S0-BYF-753

The Juice Lady's

REMEDIES

FOR DIABETES

CHERIE CALBOM, MSN, CN

SILOAM

Most CHARISMA HOUSE BOOK GROUP products are available at special quantity discounts for bulk purchase for sales promotions, premiums, fund-raising, and educational needs. For details, write Charisma House Book Group, 600 Rinehart Road, Lake Mary, Florida 32746, or telephone (407) 333-0600.

THE JUICE LADY'S REMEDIES FOR DIABETES
by Cherie Calbom
Published by Siloam
Charisma Media/Charisma House Book Group
600 Rinehart Road
Lake Mary, Florida 32746
www.charismahouse.com

Cover design by Justin Evans

Visit the author's website at www.juiceladycherie.com.

Library of Congress Cataloguing-in-Publication Data:
An application to register this book for cataloging has been submitted to the Library of Congress.
International Standard Book Number: 978-1-62998-648-7
E-book ISBN: 978-1-62998-754-5

Portions of this book were previously published as *The Juice Lady's Living Foods Revolution* by Siloam, ISBN 978-1-61638-363-3, copyright © 2011; *The Juice Lady's Weekend Weight Loss Diet* by Siloam, ISBN

978-1-61638-656-6, copyright © 2011; *The Juice Lady's Big Book of Juices and Green Smoothies by Siloam*, ISBN 978-1-62136-030-8, copyright © 2013; *The Juice Lady's Remedies for Asthma and Allergies*, ISBN 978-1-62136-601-0, copyright © 2014; and *The Juice Lady's Remedies for Thyroid Disorders*, ISBN 978-1-62998-204-5, copyright © 2015.

publisher nor the author assumes any responsibility for errors or for changes that occur after publication.

This publication is translated in Spanish under the title *Los remedios para la Diabetes de la Dama de los Jugos*, copyright © 2016 by Cherie Calbom, MSN, CN, published by Casa Creación, a Charisma Media company. All rights reserved.

16 17 18 19 20 — 987654321
Printed in the United States of America

CONTENTS

INTRODUCTION

I BECAME KNOWN AS "the Juice Lady" on TV and in print because of a serendipitous request from the owners of the Juiceman company. I was living in Seattle, Washington, completing graduate school at Bastyr University (a school of natural medicine), when another graduate student and I were asked to write a booklet containing juice recipes and nutrition information to accompany the Juiceman Juicer. One thing led to another, and before long I was traveling around the country almost weekly as the Juice Lady, teaching people how to create nutritious juices that are guaranteed to renew health and vitality.

Even before I decided to pursue my master's degree in nutrition science, I had a passionate personal interest in the benefits of high-quality nutrition because it was juicing, detoxing, and eating whole organic foods that had brought me back to full health not only once, but twice. (Read my story in chapter 1.) Now I want nothing more than to bring other people along with me on the journey to full life.

In this book I want to introduce you to the special benefits of juicing to help you prevent diabetes or to improve your health if you have already been diagnosed with diabetes.

Many people need this information today. Diabetes affects more than 29.1 million people in the United States, more than 9.3 percent of the population (people of all ages). Of that number, 21 million people have been diagnosed with the disease, and 8.1 million people (or 27.8 percent of people with diabetes) have not yet been diagnosed.[1]

Diabetes is actually a group of diseases (including both type 1 and type 2, as well as others) marked by high levels of blood glucose caused from problems in how insulin is produced, how insulin works, or both. Diabetics may develop serious complications, including heart disease, stroke, kidney failure, limb loss, blindness, and premature death.[2]

Thanks to better treatments, diabetics are living longer and have a better quality of life than ever before. Healthy food choices are an especially important part of any successful treatment program. In this book we will explore how food choices—especially "juiceable" foods—can help slow down the progress and calm the symptoms of the disease.

Diabetes is a serious disease, but it does not need to be an irreversible life sentence. You can look forward to a long and happy life after a diagnosis of diabetes—if you make specific changes to your lifestyle. I have worked with many people who have been able to manage their diabetes with diet alone. After following my recommendations for thirty days, many people have reported that their blood sugar returned to normal, and a significant percentage no longer needed medication as long as they followed the diet.

Are you ready for something better? It's time for you to learn to make highly nutritious juices in your own kitchen. Juices and smoothies made from fresh vegetables, low-sugar fruits, and other foods can help you regain your health and vitality—and keep you healthy for the rest of your life. Let fresh and nutritious juices, smoothies, and living foods become your insurance against the multifaceted threats of diabetes to the healthy functioning of your body.

Fresh is best.

Why go to the trouble of making your own juice? Why not just buy it? After all, stores are now stocked with a growing array of juices and other beverages made from organic, natural ingredients.

The primary reason is that you simply cannot get complete nutritional benefits from juice that is not freshly made, regardless of how carefully it was bottled and stored. Too many of the vitamins and other nutrients are lost or altered in juice that is not fresh, even when it has been produced from the finest ingredients. Many prepackaged juices have been pasteurized, meaning that high heat has been applied to the processing, which kills vitamins, enzymes, and biophotons.

Another obvious reason is that your choices will be limited to whatever sells best. Only juice recipes that are commercially viable will be manufactured and sold at your local store. If you learn to make your own juices, smoothies, and other beverages, you will be able to pick and choose based not only on your personal health needs but also on your taste preferences. You may never buy juice again once your taste buds sample their first sip of one of the juices in this book. Take a quick look at the last chapter, where you will find recipes using ingredients more varied and numerous than you will ever be able to try with store-bought juice. After a while you will be creating your own special combinations of yummy, fresh ingredients.

Your digestive system will be able to absorb the nutrition quickly—without raising your blood sugar too much—so that it can enter your bloodstream and begin to achieve its complex healing work. The vitamins, minerals, enzymes, phytochemicals, biophotons, and more—all extracted from nature's own containers—will make you feel healthier almost instantly.

To focus on the nutritional needs of people with diabetes (or prediabetes), I have specially selected from my always-growing collection of recipes. There is a reason for every one of my choices and combinations, and I have tried to balance tastes and other personal preferences with the changing health needs of people like you who don't have all day to work in the garden or stand at the kitchen counter but who want to zero in on top-notch nutrition that is both healthful and healing.

"Juice"—both a noun and a verb

Anybody can learn to juice. To get started, all you need is a good juicer. (On my website, www.juiceladycherie.com, you will find recommendations for juicers.) Skim the recipes in this book until one catches your eye. Stock your refrigerator and pantry shelves and plug in your juicer. Within minutes you will take your first sip. Later in the day find another recipe and give it a try. After a couple of weeks of your new routine I know you will be feeling better. Your sluggishness will disappear, and you will be able to make other important lifestyle changes. Before long you may be able to say no to extreme medical interventions, and your troubling (even debilitating) symptoms of diabetes will be a thing of the past.

Here's to your health—as I raise another tall glass of freshest juice! I am a living testimony to its benefits.

Chapter 1

MY STORY

Y LIFE CHANGED years ago when I discovered the healing power of freshly made juice as well as raw, whole foods. I'd like to share my story with you.

I had been sick for a couple years and just kept getting worse. I was sitting by the window one day in my father's home staring at the snow-topped mountains in the distance. It was early June, and the weather was beautiful. I wished I had the strength to just walk around the block. But I was too sick and tired—I could barely walk around the house.

"Will I ever be well again?" I wondered. I'd had to quit my job when I turned thirty because I had chronic fatigue syndrome and fibromyalgia. They made me so sick I couldn't work. I felt as though I had a never-ending flu. Constantly feverish with swollen glands and perennially lethargic, I was also in constant pain. My body ached as though I'd been bounced around in a washing machine.

I had moved back to my father's home in Colorado to try to recover. But not one doctor had a recommendation for what I should do to facilitate healing. So I went to some health food stores and browsed around, talked with employees, and read a few books. I decided that everything I'd been doing—eating fast food, having granola for dinner, and not eating vegetables—was tearing down my health rather than healing my body. I read about juicing and whole foods, and it made sense to me. So I bought a juicer and designed a program I could follow.

I juiced and ate a nearly perfect diet of live and whole foods for three months. There were ups and downs throughout. I had days on which I felt encouraged that I was making some progress but other days on which I felt worse. The latter were discouraging and made me wonder if health was the elusive dream. No one told me about detox reactions, which was what I was experiencing. I was obviously very toxic, and my body was cleansing away all that stuff that had made me sick. This caused the not-so-good days in the midst of the promising ones.

But one morning I woke up early—early for me, which was around 8:00 a.m.—without an alarm sounding off. I felt as if someone had given me a new body in the night. I had so much energy I actually wanted to go jogging! What had happened? This new sensation of health seemed to have appeared with the morning sun. But actually my body had been healing all along; the healing simply had not manifested until that day.

What a wonderful sense of being alive! I looked and felt completely renewed. With my juicer in tow and a new lifestyle fully embraced, I returned to Southern California a couple weeks later to finish writing my first book. For nearly a year I enjoyed great health and more energy and stamina than I'd ever remembered.

But just ahead was a shattering event.

Death too near

July fourth was a beautiful day like so many others in Southern California. I celebrated the holiday with friends that evening at a backyard barbecue. When the evening got cool, we put on jackets and watched fireworks light up the night sky. I had been house-sitting for some vacationing friends who lived in a lovely neighborhood nearby, and I returned just before midnight. Soon I was snug in bed.

I woke up shivering some time later. "Why is it so cold?" I

wondered, as I rolled over to see the clock; it was 3:00 a.m. That's when I noticed that the door to the backyard was open. "Wonder how that happened?" I thought, as I began to get up to close and lock it. That's when I noticed a man crouched in the shadows of the corner of the room—a shirtless young guy in shorts. I blinked twice, trying to deny what I was seeing. Instead of running, he leaped off the floor and ran toward me. He pulled a pipe from his shorts and began attacking me, beating me repeatedly over the head and yelling, "Now you are dead!" We fought—or I should say I tried to defend myself and grab the pipe. It finally flew out of his hands. That's when he choked me to unconsciousness. I felt life leaving my body.

"This is it, the end of my life," I thought. I felt sad for the people who loved me and how they would feel about this tragic event. Then I felt my spirit leave in a sensation of popping out of my body and floating upward. Suddenly everything was peaceful and still. I sensed I was traveling at what seemed like the speed of light through black space. I saw what looked like lights twinkling in the distance. But all of a sudden I was back in my body, outside the house, clinging to a fence at the end of the dog run. I don't know how I got there. I screamed for help with all the breath I had. My third scream took all my strength. I felt it would be my last. Each time I screamed, I passed out and landed on the cement. I then had to pull myself up again. But this time a neighbor heard me and sent her husband to help. Within a short time I was on my way to the hospital.

Lying on a cold gurney at 4:30 a.m., chilled to the bone, in and out of consciousness, I tried to assess my injuries. When I finally looked at my right hand, I almost passed out again. My ring finger was barely hanging on by a small piece of skin. My hand was split open, and I could see deep inside. The next thing

I knew, I was being wheeled off to surgery. Later I learned that I had suffered serious injuries to my head, neck, back, and right hand, with multiple head wounds and part of my scalp torn from my head. I also incurred numerous cracked teeth that required several root canals and crowns months later.

My right hand sustained the most severe injuries, with two knuckles crushed to mere bone fragments that had to be held together by three metal pins. Six months after the attack I still couldn't use it. The cast I wore—with bands holding up the ring finger, which had almost been torn from my hand, and various odd-shaped molded parts—looked like something from a science-fiction movie. I felt and looked worse than hopeless, with a shaved top of my head, totally red and swollen eyes, a gash on my face, a useless right hand, terrorizing fear, and barely enough energy to get dressed in the morning. I was an emotional wreck.

I couldn't sleep at night—not even a minute. It was torturous. Never mind that I was staying with a cousin and his family. There was no need to worry about safety from a practical point of view, but that made no difference emotionally. I'd lie in bed all night and stare at the ceiling or the bedroom door. I had five lights that I kept on all night. I'd try to read, but my eyes would sting. I could sleep for only a little while during the day.

But the worst part was the pain in my soul that nearly took my breath away. All the emotional pain of the attack combined with the pain and trauma of my past felt like an emotional tsunami. My past had been riddled with loss, trauma, and anxiety. My brother had died when I was two. My mother had died of cancer when I was six. I couldn't remember much about her death—the memories seemed blocked. But my cousin said I fainted at her funeral. That told me the impact was huge.

I had lived for the next three years with my father and

maternal grandparents. But Grandpa John, the love of my life, died when I was nine. The loss was immeasurable. Four years later my father was involved in a very tragic situation that would take far too long to discuss here, but it was horrific. He was no longer in my daily life. I felt terrified about my future. My grandmother was eighty-six. I had no idea how many more years she would live. The next year I moved to Oregon to live with an aunt and uncle until I graduated from high school.

Wrapped in my soul was a huge amount of anguish and pain with all sorts of triggers for emotional and binge eating. I know firsthand about eating-disorder behavior—binge eating and then not eating anything for a few days. I know what it is to get triggered emotionally and be clueless as to what set off an eating binge. Food is immediate comfort. It's often the first thing we turn to. It was for me. But not wanting to gain a lot of weight, I would then avoid food for a day or two after binge eating.

To heal physically, mentally, and emotionally after the attack took every ounce of my will, faith, and trust in God. I did deep spiritual work, sought alternative medical help, took extra vitamins and minerals, resumed vegetable juicing, and experienced the emotional release of healing prayer and numerous detox programs. I met a nutritionally minded physician who had healed his own slow-mending broken bones with lots of vitamin-mineral IVs. He gave me similar IVs. Juicing, cleansing, nutritional supplements, a nearly perfect diet, prayer, and physical therapy helped my bones and other injuries heal.

After following this regimen for about nine months, what my hand surgeon said was impossible became a reality—a fully restored, fully functional hand. He had told me that it wasn't possible to put in plastic knuckles because of the hand's poor condition and that I'd never use my right hand again. But my knuckles did indeed re-form—primarily due to prayer—and the function of my hand returned. A day came when he told me I was completely healed, and though he admitted he didn't believe in miracles, he said, "You're the closest thing I've seen to one."

The healing of my hand was indeed a miracle! I had a useful hand again, and my career in writing was not over as I had thought it would be. My inner wounds were more severe than the physical devastation, and they were the hardest to heal. Nevertheless, they mended too. I experienced healing from the painful memories and trauma of the attack and the wounds from the past through prayer, laying on of hands, and deep emotional healing work. I called the ladies who prayed for me around their kitchen table week after week until my soul was healed. I call them my *kitchen angels*. I cried endless buckets of tears that had been pent up in my soul. I desperately needed the release. Forgiveness and letting go came in stages and proved to be an integral part of my total healing. I had to be honest about what I really felt and be willing to face the pain and toxic emotions confined inside, and then let them go. Finally, after a very long journey, I felt free. Eventually I could even celebrate the Fourth of July without fear.

Today I know more peace and health than I ever thought would be possible. I have experienced what it is to feel whole—complete, not damaged, broken, wounded, or impaired— truly healed and restored in body, soul, and spirit. And I'm not plagued with emotional eating anymore.

I have learned that my purpose is to love people to life through my writing and nutritional information and to help them find their way to health and healing. If I could recover from all that had happened to me, they can too. No matter what anyone is facing, there is hope. I want you to know that you are loved, and

I send you my love between the lines of this book and with the juice and raw-food recipes. There is hope for you.

Now this book is about diabetes, which I have never had although I was diagnosed with hypoglycemia (low blood sugar). But so much of what I have learned applies to diabetics. Weight loss and maintenance? I have you covered. Need to know more about sugar? Yes, I can help you with that too. Want to know how to stabilize your blood sugar? I've helped many people accomplish that.

You do not have to continue suffering the results of stress and exhaustion or the uncomfortable effects of diabetes medications. No matter what challenges you face, there are answers that will heal your body, mind, and spirit. There's a purpose for your life, just as there was for mine. You need to be strong and well to complete your purpose. You can be greatly served by a positive mind and an optimistic attitude. With God's help and the latest nutritional data in this book, you can facilitate abundant health, learn the right way to live your life to the fullest, and finish well.

Chapter 2

DIABETES AND YOU

G OSH, I'M SO thirsty all the time! And then I have to run to the restroom so often."

"I'm hungry too. It doesn't make sense. I'm eating like a horse and yet losing weight."

"So, so, so tired...even when I get enough sleep."

"It's been a tough year for infections—can't seem to get on top of them."

"What's going on? I thought I needed new glasses, but I guess I don't."

"It just seems I'm more irritable than usual."

Perhaps after months or years of noticing unpleasant symptoms,[1] you finally made an appointment with your family physician. (It's possible you had no symptoms at all and that the disease was discovered during routine testing.) Now you know that, yes, you really do have diabetes, and you are grappling with the implications for your future and your whole way of life. It's not easy; regardless of the fact that thousands of other people are living with the same disease—some possibly within your own family—this is *you* we're talking about, not a name in an appointment book or a number in the statistics.

For you and for others, what does this beast called "diabetes" look like, anyway?

Primary Types of Diabetes

There are two primary types of diabetes.[2]

Type 1 diabetes

"Type 1 diabetes was previously called insulin-dependent diabetes mellitus or juvenile-onset diabetes. Although disease onset can occur at any age, the peak age for diagnosis is in the mid-teens. Type 1 diabetes develops when the cells in the pancreas that produce the hormone insulin, known as the beta cells, in the pancreas are destroyed. The destruction is initiated or mediated by the body's immune system and limits or completely eliminates the production and secretion of insulin, the hormone that is required to lower blood glucose levels. To survive, people with type 1 diabetes must have insulin delivered by injection or a pump. In adults, type 1 diabetes accounts for approximately 5% of all diagnosed cases of diabetes. There is no known way to prevent type 1 diabetes. Several clinical trials for preventing type 1 diabetes are currently in progress with additional studies being planned."

I do have my own theories, though. I believe that many people could prevent even type 1 diabetes by eliminating all refined sugar and refined carbohydrates.

Type 2 diabetes

"Type 2 diabetes was previously called non–insulin-dependent diabetes mellitus or adult-onset diabetes because the peak age of onset is usually later than it is for type 1 diabetes. In adults, type 2 diabetes accounts for about 90% to 95% of all diagnosed cases of diabetes. Type 2 diabetes usually begins with insulin resistance, a disorder in which the cells primarily within the muscles, liver, and fat tissue, do not use insulin properly. As the need for insulin rises, the beta cells in the pancreas gradually lose the ability to produce sufficient quantities of the hormone. The role of insulin resistance as opposed to beta cell dysfunction differs among individuals, with some having primarily insulin resistance and only a minor defect in insulin secretion and others having slight insulin resistance and primarily a lack of insulin secretion.

"The risk for developing type 2 diabetes is associated with older age, obesity, family history of diabetes, history of gestational diabetes, impaired glucose metabolism, physical inactivity, and race/ethnicity. African Americans, Hispanics/Latinos, American Indians, some Asians, and Native Hawaiians or other Pacific Islanders are at particularly high risk for type 2 diabetes and its complications. Type 2 diabetes in children and adolescents, although uncommon, is being diagnosed more frequently among American Indians, African Americans, Hispanics/Latinos, Asians, and Pacific Islanders."

Other Types of Diabetes

Gestational diabetes

"Gestational diabetes is a form of glucose intolerance diagnosed during the second or third trimester of pregnancy. During pregnancy, increasing blood glucose levels increase the risk for both mother and fetus and require treatment to reduce problems for the mother and infant. Treatment may include diet, regular physical activity, or insulin. Shortly after pregnancy, 5% to 10% of women with gestational diabetes continue to have high blood glucose levels and are diagnosed as having diabetes, usually type 2. The risk factors for gestational diabetes are similar to those for type 2 diabetes. The occurrence of gestational diabetes itself is a risk factor for developing recurrent gestational diabetes with future pregnancies and subsequent development of type 2 diabetes. Also, the children of women who had gestational diabetes during pregnancies may be at risk of developing obesity and diabetes."

Additional types

"Other types of diabetes, such as maturity-onset diabetes of youth or latent autoimmune diabetes in adults, among others, are caused by specific genetic conditions or from surgery, medications, infections, pancreatic disease, or other illnesses. Such types of diabetes account for 1% to 5% of all diagnosed cases."

Prediabetes

"Prediabetes is a condition in which individuals have high blood glucose or hemoglobin A1C levels but not high enough to be classified as diabetes. People with prediabetes have an increased risk of developing type 2 diabetes, heart disease, and stroke, but not everyone with prediabetes will progress to diabetes. The Diabetes Prevention Program, a large prevention study of people at high risk for diabetes, showed that lifestyle intervention that resulted in weight loss and increased physical activity in this population can prevent or delay type 2 diabetes and in some cases return blood glucose levels to within the normal range. Other international studies have shown similar results."[3]

Metabolic syndrome

Metabolic syndrome is a condition characterized by obesity (with most of the weight being carried around the waist), high blood pressure, high triglycerides (fats in the blood), low HDL (also known as "good cholesterol"), and impaired metabolism of glucose. Metabolic syndrome increases the risk of developing diabetes significantly.[4]

WHAT IS DIABETES?

Diabetes is a metabolic disorder characterized by excessive glucose (sugar) in a person's blood. The body is unable to use it properly, so it must excrete it in the urine (along with water). Either the pancreas does not produce enough of the hormone insulin or the body cells cannot react properly to insulin. (Insulin is like the "key" that lets glucose into the cells of the body, providing energy. Much of our necessary glucose comes from digesting carbohydrates.)

Lowering Blood-Glucose Levels

If you have been diagnosed with diabetes, lowering and stabilizing your blood-glucose levels will be yours and your doctor's goal. Thus the successful treatment and management of your condition may include oral medication (until you can stabilize your blood sugar with diet and exercise), insulin, if needed, and diet. Exercise also plays an important role. Many people with diabetes need to lose weight, and some must learn to control their cholesterol count and blood pressure.

A healthy eating plan can go a long way toward achieving the goals of lowering glucose levels in the blood, losing weight, and controlling cholesterol and blood pressure numbers. The rest of this book will help you figure out how to make the best possible eating choices for your personal situation.

Overall you should eat smaller portions than you may have been used to eating. You will need to learn what a serving size is for different foods and how many servings you need in a meal. It is important to eat less fat. Choose fewer high-fat foods and use less fat for cooking. You especially want to limit foods that are high in saturated fats or trans fat, such as fatty cuts of meat, fried foods, whole milk and dairy products made from whole milk, "high carb" baked goods (cakes, candy, cookies, crackers, pies), salad dressings, lard, shortening, stick margarine, and nondairy creamers.[5] And you want to eat a low-carb diet, eliminating sweets and refined carbohydrates. You also want to avoid fruit except for low-sugar fruit such as berries, lemons, limes, and green apples.

By eating less fat (along with no sugar) you may be able to reverse insulin resistance. A review of studies about bariatric surgery (surgery offered to people who are morbidly obese to reduce the size of their stomach and bypass a portion of the small intestine) proves this point. In many cases type 2 diabetes was reversed within days of the surgery—before much weight loss could have been achieved. Apparently the improvement results from the sudden decrease of triglycerides and fatty acids in the bloodstream, along with an immediate reduction of fats in liver and muscle cells.[6]

You will need to concentrate on eating more fiber, found not only in whole-grain foods such as oatmeal; brown, black, and red rice; quinoa; millet; buckwheat; and kamut but also in a variety of low-sugar fruits and vegetables. Eat plenty of veggies from the groups below:

- Dark green veggies (e.g., broccoli, spinach, brussels sprouts)

- Orange veggies (e.g., carrots, sweet potatoes, pumpkin, winter squash)

- Beans and peas (e.g., black beans, garbanzo beans, kidney beans, pinto beans, split peas, lentils)

At the same time you will need to avoid foods and beverages that are high in sugar, such as sweetened drinks (including juices that are not 100 percent fruit-based, sodas, and tea or coffee sweetened with sugar). You should use less salt in cooking and at the table. Limit your consumption of foods that are high in salt, such as canned and packaged soups, canned vegetables, pickles, and processed meats.[7]

About those carbs

You've probably heard of "glycemic index" and "glycemic load," not to mention "counting carbs." What do these terms mean?

Both glycemic index and glycemic load concern carbohydrates (carbs), which are one of the main types of nutrients in the human diet. Carbs with a simple chemical structure are called "sugars," and they are found naturally in foods such as sugar, fruit juice, milk, yogurt, honey, refined flour products, sodas, maple syrup, brown sugar, agave, and milk products. "Complex carbs" (think starches and fiber) are found in whole grains, cereal grasses, vegetables, fruit, nuts, seeds, and legumes.

LEGUMES

Legumes (beans, lentils, dried peas) are packed with nutrition, including protein, calcium, vitamins, and minerals. And they are very cheap. When cooked right, they are delicious. They can also be sprouted. Legumes offer a lot of health benefits. They help prevent food cravings, metabolic syndrome, type 2 diabetes, and obesity. That's because the outer casing of legumes, which is high fiber, slows down the rate at 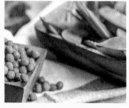 which sugar enters your blood stream. Legumes also protect the body against cancer and heart disease. Further, they provide lots of protein for energy.

Your digestive system changes the carbohydrates you consume into glucose, a type of sugar that your body uses for energy. Because simple carbs are more quickly digested and absorbed than complex ones, simple carbs can raise your blood-glucose levels faster and higher. People with diabetes must manage their blood-glucose levels. High blood glucose can damage tissues and organs, leading to heart disease, blindness, kidney failure, and other problems over time.

Glycemic index and glycemic load

The glycemic index (GI) has been developed to show how the carbs in different foods raise blood sugar. White bread, for example, has a higher glycemic index than whole-grain bread, which contains more complex carbs. But it's not just the *types* of carbs that matter. The *more* carbs you eat, the more your blood sugar rises.

That's why researchers came up with the concept of glycemic load. It captures both the types of carbs in a food and the amount of carbs in a serving. Essentially it shows how a portion of a particular food affects your blood sugar. Many things affect the glycemic load (GL), including food processing, how ripe a fruit is, how a food is prepared, and how long it's been stored. Because it's calculated based on GI (as a percentage) multiplied by the carb count in an average serving, GL can be a much more useful number to go by. See appendix B for more information.

Glycemic index and glycemic load aren't things you'll see on a label, so they're not easy to determine. But you can learn the basics from the online publications of organizations such as the American Diabetes Association.[8]

Meats and fats don't have a glycemic index because they do not contain carbohydrates. But in order to balance the GI of your meals and snacks, you must choose your other foods purposefully. For the most part, meal planning with the glycemic index in mind means choosing low- to medium-GI foods, and if you consume something with a high GI, you should be sure to choose low GI foods to balance it out.

Here is a basic guide that I've adapted from the American Diabetes Association:[9]

Low GI foods (55 or less)

- One hundred percent stone-ground whole wheat or pumpernickel bread
- Oatmeal (rolled or steel-cut), oat bran, muesli
- Pasta, barley, bulgar
- Sweet potato, corn, yam, lima/butter beans, peas, legumes, lentils
- Low-sugar fruits, non-starchy vegetables and carrots

Medium GI (56–69)

- Whole wheat, rye, and pita bread
- Quick oats
- Brown, wild or basmati rice, couscous

High GI (70 or more)

- White bread or bagel
- Corn flakes, puffed rice, bran flakes, instant oatmeal
- Short-grain white rice, rice pasta, macaroni and cheese from mix
- Russet potato, pumpkin
- Pretzels, rice cakes, popcorn, saltine crackers

- Melons and pineapple

As I mentioned before, some of the factors that can affect the actual GI include ripeness and storage time, the amount of processing and/or the cooking method, and variations in the type of an item chosen. For example, the more ripe a fruit or vegetable is, the higher the GI will be. The longer a food is cooked (and thus the softer and more easily absorbed), the higher the GI will be. The Italians have it right—al dente pasta is better than mushy pasta.[10]

In general raw and fresh vegetables rank very low on the glycemic index, and they also carry a low glycemic load because they are loaded with fiber. Cooking them softens the fiber and causes the carbs to be more readily available, which is why the GI number for cooked vegetables is higher than for the raw form of the same food.

DAILY CARB INTAKE

"The American Diabetes Foundation...reports that a daily carbohydrate intake of 135 to 180 grams per day is a typical goal for diabetics. That works out to 45 to 60 grams of carbohydrates per meal, leaving ample room for sensible portions of fruits."[11]

I would add that I've found it best to make that low-sugar fruit only.

The bottom line: Though carbohydrate management is not the whole solution to diabetes, knowing the GI for a variety of foods will help you eat smart and achieve better blood-glucose levels.

Insulin Resistance Self-Test

Insulin resistance is a condition in which cells fail to respond to the normal actions of the hormone insulin. The body produces insulin, but the cells in the body become resistant to insulin and are unable to use it as effectively. If you have insulin resistance, you may be gaining weight and feel tired and hungry. The afternoon "blahs" may occur more often than not. You may be thirstier, or you may wake up at night to go to the bathroom. These symptoms are some of the most common associated with insulin resistance. More than eighty million Americans suffer from insulin resistance, also known as "syndrome X." Many do not even know they have it, so they are probably unaware of the health problems associated with it. Those with insulin resistance have a greater risk of diabetes, hypertension, heart disease, obesity, high cholesterol, breast cancer, and polycystic ovarian syndrome (PCOS). Take the self-test and see where you stand[12]:

1. What is your Body Mass Index (BMI)? (Weight divided by your height squared.)

   (a) Below 25

   (b) Between 25–28

   (c) Above 28

2. Most of your weight is carried…

   (a) On your hips, thighs, and buttocks

   (b) In a small bump on your tummy

   (c) All around the stomach area

3. You tend to put on weight fast:

   (a) No, never

   (b) Yes, but only if I eat more than usual

   (c) Yes, even without excessive overeating

4. When you follow a healthy eating program, you:

   (a) Never follow a diet because you're not overweight

   (b) Lose a little if it's followed to the letter

   (c) Never have success losing weight even when you're
       "strict"

5. Do you or a member of your family have diabetes,
   heart issues such as high cholesterol or high blood
   pressure, or gout?

   (a) No

   (b) Yes, at least one of these apply to me or my family

   (c) Yes, more than one of these apply to me or my family

6. If you are a female, do you have polycystic ovarian
   syndrome?

   (a) No, not that I am aware (or not female)

   (b) Yes

7. Do you suffer with fluid retention in general?

   (a) No

   (b) At certain times of the month: e.g., premenstrual,
       or if I've been walking a lot

   (c) Often notice my feet, ankles, legs, or fingers are
       swollen

8. If you are a female, do you suffer from premenstrual tension, including food cravings and mood swings?

   (a) No (or not female)

   (b) Some months, depending

   (c) Every month, and it's pretty awful

9. Do you suffer from depression?

   (a) No

   (b) Unsure, or have in the past suffered from depression

   (c) Yes

10. Do you experience frequent food cravings, especially for sugary or starchy foods?

    (a) No

    (b) Sometimes

    (c) All the time!

11. Do your food cravings, especially for sweet or starchy foods, occur later in the day, especially in the late afternoon and evening?

    (a) No (or no cravings)

    (b) Sometimes

    (c) Most of the time!

12. Do you suffer from mood swings?

    (a) No

    (b) Sometimes

    (c) All the time!

13. Are you usually tired, or do you suffer from fatigue in the afternoon or early evening?

   (a) No

   (b) Sometimes

   (c) Most days!

14. Have you experienced excessive thirst and frequent urination?

   (a) No

   (b) Yes, at least one of the above

   (c) Both of the above!

Mostly (a)

The chances are that you do not have insulin resistance. These questions are not the only criteria for diagnosing insulin resistance, and often a combination of factors (including blood tests) will enable a diagnosis of insulin resistance to be made. You may want to keep supporting your blood-sugar levels as a preventative measure by continuing to juice veggies, eat healthy foods, and exercise.

Mostly (b)

You may have insulin resistance or be at risk of developing insulin resistance. These questions are not the only criteria for diagnosing insulin resistance, and often a combination of factors (including blood tests) will enable a diagnosis of insulin resistance to be made. If you would like more information, contact your local dietician or health care provider. You may consider trying to balance your sugar levels naturally.

Mostly (c)

You are at high risk for insulin resistance and may already be insulin resistant. These questions are not the only criteria for diagnosing insulin resistance, and often a combination of factors (including blood tests) will enable a diagnosis of insulin resistance to be made. It is recommended that you speak with your health-care provider about insulin resistance. You also need to balance your blood-sugar levels. You may also need help to lose weight in a healthy way and may want to sign up for nutrition counseling.

Chapter 3

THE IMPORTANCE OF
LOSING WEIGHT

FOR PEOPLE WITH prediabetes, weight loss and other life-style modifications can decrease the risk of developing full-blown diabetes by as much as 58 percent.[1] For people who have already progressed to diabetes, about half of the men and 70 percent of the women are obese at the time of diagnosis.[2] According to WebMD, "If you're overweight and have type 2 diabetes, you will lower your blood sugar, improve your health, and feel better if you lose some of your extra pounds."[3] Dropping even 10 or 15 pounds offers health perks such as lower blood pressure; better cholesterol levels; less stress on your hips, knees, ankles, and feet; more energy; and improved mood.[4]

But you know how hard it is to lose weight and keep it off. Voluntary, intentional weight loss is never easy, and if anybody tries to tell you that his amazing new product will make it effortless, you have learned (probably the hard way) that it's not true. And yet, for the sake of your health and longevity, you must try to achieve and maintain a normal weight. For diabetics, it can be an especially vicious circle: weight gain can lead to insulin resistance, and taking supplementary insulin can cause more weight gain.

Why do diabetics gain and retain weight so easily? Type 1 diabetes requires the regular administration of insulin, and so does type 2 diabetes if it cannot be controlled otherwise. If you take insulin, you are adding a hormone to your body that regulates the absorption of glucose by the cells of your body. A dose of insulin allows glucose to enter your cells, and glucose levels in your blood drop accordingly. This is good. But it's easy to take in more calories than you need, especially if you have a sedentary lifestyle. That means your cells will be getting more glucose than they need——and what they don't use gets stored as fat.[5]

The usual advice applies: count calories, choose foods carefully, limit your portion sizes, skip seconds, and drink lots of water. However, don't try to cut calories by skipping meals. This can cause your blood-sugar level to dip if you don't adjust your insulin dose, and you will be tempted to make up later for "starving" yourself. You should take your insulin exactly as directed because the risks associated with reducing the dosage for the sake of weight loss are significant. You may decide to inquire about other diabetes medications. Some of them promote weight loss and allow you to take less insulin.[6]

The importance of physical activity cannot be overemphasized. Exercise works wonders for both your metabolism and your mood.

Tips for Weight-Loss Success

Cut your calories. Most people lose weight when they embark on a healthy eating and vegetable-juicing program because they stop craving junk food and high-carb foods, which helps cut a lot of calories. But make sure you shave off at least one hundred calories from your daily caloric intake. All long-term weight studies ever done in which people kept the weight off for more than two years showed this simple strategy. It's very easy to do, and one hundred calories is such a small amount your body won't be able to tell you're on a diet. This way your metabolism doesn't slow down, and you naturally lose weight. But don't worry if you shave off more than one hundred calories a day, as you probably will. Your metabolism should not slow down because this style of eating is replete with living nutrients such as vitamins, enzymes, and biophotons that rev up your metabolism.

Eat breakfast. If you think skipping breakfast will cut a bunch of calories from your diet and speed your weight loss, you're mistaken. People who skip breakfast usually eat more for lunch because they're so hungry, and they usually snack more throughout the day. Start your day with a power breakfast that begins with a glass of raw veggie juice and/or a green or nut smoothie. Many people say they just aren't hungry anymore after drinking an energizing glass of veggie juice or a green smoothie. That may be all you want, but if you're still hungry, follow with some protein such as raw nuts or seeds, raw veggie dip and fresh vegetables, a vegetable omelet, or a bowl of old-fashioned, steel-cut oatmeal. In a study of people who dropped at least thirty pounds, 78 percent said they ate breakfast.[7] Make sure you eat something within an hour of rising. This habit will boost your metabolism by 10 percent.

Eat healthy snacks. Each day, if you work outside the home, pack healthy snacks in small containers or plastic bags to take with you and keep in your purse, briefcase, or an insulated tote. If you always have healthy, diet-friendly snacks such as fresh veggies, low-sugar fruit, raw nuts, or seeds on hand, you'll be less tempted to raid the vending machine or grab a few pieces of candy from a coworker's dish. And you won't go home ravenously hungry and eat half a bag of chips or cookies before diner.

Drink purified water. The next time you feel hungry, drink a glass of purified water. You may not need to eat afterward. Since the hormones in our intestinal tract that tell us we're hungry are very similar to the hormones that let us know we're thirsty, it's often hard to distinguish hunger from thirst. Therefore, we reach for food when we should be reaching for water. Your hunger pangs could be your body's cry for H2O. Water is essential for burning calories. People who drink eight or more glasses of water a day burn more calories than those who drink fewer.[8] If you don't like the taste of plain water, add fresh lemon or cranberry juice. I like lemon and ginger juice added to my water. You may also want to invest in a good water purifier. It's amazing how that improves the taste and purity of the water, and pure water contributes to better health.

CRANBERRY WATER

To make cranberry water, start with an 8-ounce glass of purified water. Add 1–2 tablespoons of unsweetened cranberry juice (just juice, nothing added) or 1 teaspoon of cranberry concentrate. Adjust cranberry juice to taste. You may add a few drops of stevia, as desired.

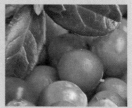

Add some coconut oil to your diet. Coconut oil is a healthy weight-loss ingredient. Not only does it boost metabolism and speed weight loss, there is also evidence that suggests that adding a small amount of coconut oil into one's daily diet can help lower cholesterol and improve conditions such as diabetes, chronic fatigue syndrome, IBS, Crohn's disease and other digestive disorders. It can also enhance thyroid production as well as increase overall energy.

GARLIC AND WEIGHT LOSS

When it comes to weight loss, garlic appears to be a miracle food. A team of doctors at Israel's Tel Hashomer Hospital conducted a test on rats to find out how garlic can prevent diabetes and heart attacks, and they found an interesting side effect—none of the rats given allicin (a compound in garlic) gained weight.[9]

Garlic is a known appetite suppressant. The strong odor of garlic stimulates the satiety center in the brain, thereby reducing feelings of hunger. It also increases the brain's sensitivity to leptin, a hormone produced by fat cells that controls appetite. Further, garlic stimulates the nervous system to release hormones that speed up metabolic rate such as adrenaline. This means a greater ability to burn calories. More calories burned means less weight gained—a terrific correlation.

Go low glycemic. Low-glycemic diet plans, also known as low carb, are popular for a reason—they get results. High-glycemic foods raise blood-sugar levels, cause the body to secrete excess insulin, and lead to the storage of fat. Originally developed as a tool to help diabetics manage blood sugar, the low-glycemic diet has become popular in the weight-loss market largely because it works so well. See appendix A for a list of helpful foods.

The focus of any nutrition therapy should be on glycemic control—preventing further weight gain and losing weight as needed. (Often weight loss will be achieved as a "side effect" as you eat to control your blood sugar.) According to certified dietitian and diabetes educator Marion J. Franz, "Setting realistic weight goals and aiming for moderation is generally the best approach: eating a healthful diet, being more physically active, and keeping food records along with blood glucose records so that blood glucose levels can be kept under optimal control and medications can be added or adjusted when needed. Eating fewer calories and getting regular physical activity improves blood glucose control independent of body weight and weight loss."[10]

Make one meal a day either a veggie juice or a green smoothie. If you make this meal dinner, you will really accelerate your weight-loss program. If you start your day with a glass of veggie juice, you will spark up your metabolism. You can then eat a protein breakfast. Make your meals low carb with a focus on veggies. You may also want to make one day a week a veggie juice fast.

The Benefits of Juicing

It may surprise you to learn that vegetable juice is the secret ingredient to your weight-loss success. It assists you in becoming slim and healthy due to its nutrition-packed, energizing properties. Let's face it—juicing is a lot easier than spending all your time chowing down on brussels sprouts, carrots, and broccoli. Don't get me wrong. I recommend that you eat these vegetables often, but really, just how many vegetables can you eat in a day? Thankfully you can juice and drink them with ease.

Because vegetable juice has very little sugar while offering an abundance of vitamins, minerals, enzymes, biophotons, and phytonutrients, it's incredibly helpful for weight loss. It offers what your body needs to fight cravings and do its work to keep you healthy. When you include vegetable juicing in your daily routine, not only will you eat fewer calories, but you will also gain energy.

As you may know, you can eat a whole bag of chips and still want something more to eat because you gave your body a lot of empty calories that made you feel sluggish and tired and still unsatisfied. The biggest plus of a juicing program is that it adds valuable nutrients that are easy for your body to absorb and that have a heap of health benefits at minimal caloric cost.

Whether you are just getting started juicing or you've been juicing a long time, I hope to inspire you to make vegetable juicing a daily habit—an ongoing part of your pursuit of health.

Fresh juice = vitality

Every time you pour yourself a glass of freshly made juice, picture a big vitamin-mineral cocktail with a wealth of nutrients that promote vitality. The veggies are broken down into an easily absorbable form that your body can use right away. This concentrated juice gives you energy and renews you right down to your cells. It also spares your organs all the work it takes to digest food, and that equates to more energy. It detoxifies your body as well because it's rich in antioxidants so your body doesn't have to work as hard dealing with toxic stuff.

In addition to water and easily absorbed protein and carbohydrates, juice also provides essential fatty acids, vitamins, minerals, enzymes, biophotons, and phytonutrients. And researchers are continuing to explore how various nutrients that we find in juice help the body heal and shed unwanted pounds.

The next time you make a glass of fresh juice, this is what you'll be drinking:

Protein. Did you ever consider juice to be a source of protein? Surprisingly it does offer more than you might think. We use protein to form muscles, ligaments, tendons, hair, nails, and skin. Protein is needed to create enzymes, which direct chemical reactions, and hormones that guide bodily functions. Fruits and vegetables contain lower quantities of protein than animal foods such as muscle meats and dairy products. Therefore, they are thought of as poor protein sources. But juices are concentrated forms of vegetables and fruit and so provide easily absorbed amino acids, the building blocks that make up protein. For example, sixteen ounces of carrot juice (two to three pounds of carrots) provides about five grams of protein (the equivalent of about one chicken wing or two ounces of tofu). However, vegetable protein is not complete protein so it does not provide all the amino acids your body needs. In addition to lots of dark leafy greens, you'll want to eat other protein sources such as sprouts, legumes (beans, lentils, and split peas), nuts, seeds, and whole grains. If you're not vegan, you can add pastured organic eggs and free-range, grass-fed muscle meats such as chicken, turkey, lamb, and beef along with wild-caught fish.

Carbohydrates. Vegetable juice contains carbohydrates. Carbs provide fuel for the body, which it uses for movement, heat production, and chemical reactions. The chemical bonds of carbohydrates lock in the energy a plant takes up from the sun, and this energy is released when the body burns plant food as fuel. There are three categories of carbs: simple (sugars), complex (starches and fiber), and fiber. Choose more complex carbohydrates in your diet than simple carbs. There are more simple sugars in fruit juice than in vegetable juice, which is why you should juice more vegetables and in most cases drink no more than four ounces of low-sugar fruit juice a day. *Remember to always mix fruit juice with veggie juice to dilute the sugar.* You can have more lemon and lime juice because it is very low in sugar. Both insoluble and soluble fibers are found in whole fruits and vegetables, and both types are needed for good health. Who said juice doesn't have fiber? Juice has the soluble form—pectin and gums, which are excellent for the digestive tract. Soluble fiber also helps to lower blood cholesterol levels, stabilize blood sugar, and improve good bowel bacteria.

Essential fatty acids. There is very little fat in fruit and vegetable juices, but the fats juice does contain are essential to your health. The essential fatty acids (EFAs)—linoleic and alpha-linolenic acids in particular—found in fresh juice function as components of nerve cells, cellular membranes, and hormone-like substances called prostaglandins. They are also required for energy production. You can get more essential fatty acids by eating cold-water fish, flaxseed, walnuts, or other foods.

Vitamins. Fresh juice is loaded with vitamins. Along with minerals and enzymes, vitamins take part in chemical reactions. For example, vitamin C participates in the production of collagen, one of the main types of protein found in the body. Fresh juices are excellent sources of water-soluble vitamins such as C and many of the B vitamins, as well as some fat-soluble vitamins such as vitamin E and the carotenes (known as provitamin A), which are converted to vitamin A as needed by the body, and vitamin K.

Minerals. Fresh juice is loaded with minerals. There are about two dozen minerals that your body needs to function well. Minerals, along with vitamins, are components of enzymes. They make up part of your bone, teeth, and blood tissue, and they help maintain normal cellular function. The major minerals include calcium, chloride, magnesium, phosphorus, potassium, sodium, and sulfur. Trace minerals are those needed in very small amounts. They include boron, chromium, cobalt, copper, fluoride, manganese, nickel, selenium, vanadium, and zinc. Minerals occur in inorganic forms in the soil, and plants incorporate them into their tissues by drawing them up through their tiny roots. As a part of this process, the minerals are combined with organic molecules into easily absorbable forms. Plant food is thus an excellent dietary source of minerals. Juicing is believed to provide even better mineral absorption than whole vegetables because the process of juicing makes minerals available in a highly absorbable, easily digestible form.

Enzymes. Fresh juices are chock-full of enzymes—those "living" molecules that work, with vitamins and minerals, to speed up reactions necessary for vital functions in the body. Without enzymes, we would not have life in our cells. Enzymes are prevalent in raw foods, but heat, such as cooking and pasteurization, destroys them. Most juices that are bottled, even if kept in store refrigerators, have to be pasteurized. Heat temperatures for pasteurization are required to be far above the limit of what would preserve the enzymes and vitamins. There are some "new guys on the block" that are much better choices if you aren't making your own juice. Look for juices created by high pressure processing (HPP). This type of processing uses a high level of cool pressure to destroy pathogens and ensure food safety. It extends microbiological shelf life without the application of heat. Suja is one brand that uses HPP. When you eat and drink enzyme-rich foods, these little proteins help break down food in the digestive tract, thereby sparing the pancreas, small intestine, gallbladder, and stomach—the body's enzyme producers—from overwork. This sparing action is known as the "law of adaptive secretion of digestive enzymes." When a portion of the food you eat is digested by enzymes present in the food you ingest, the body will secrete fewer of its own enzymes, thus allowing your body's energy to be shifted from digestion to other functions such as repair and rejuvenation. In other words, fresh juices require very little energy expenditure to digest. And that is one reason people who start consistently drinking fresh juice often report that they feel better and more energized right away.

Phytochemicals. Plants contain substances that protect them from disease, injury, and pollution. These substances are known as phytochemicals. *Phyto* means plant and *chemical* in this context means nutrient. There are tens of thousands of phytochemicals in the foods we eat. For example, the average tomato may contain up to ten thousand different types of phytonutrients, the most famous being lycopene. Phytochemicals give plants their color, odor, and flavor. Unlike vitamins and enzymes, they are heat stable and can withstand cooking. Researchers have found that people who eat the most fruits and vegetables, the best sources of phytonutrients, have the lowest incidence of cancer and other diseases. Drinking vegetable juices gives you these vital substances in a concentrated form.

JUICING RECOMMENDATIONS FOR DIABETICS AND PREDIABETICS

I've often heard people say they can't juice because they have diabetes. You can juice vegetables even if you have sugar-metabolism problems, but you should choose low-sugar veggies and only low-sugar fruits such as lemons, limes, green apples, berries, and cranberries. Carrots and beets are too high in sugar. You could add one or two carrots to a juice recipe or a very small beet or part of a beet, but they should be diluted with cucumber juice and dark leafy greens. You may use cranberries, berries, green apple, lemons, and limes, but other fruits are higher in sugar and should be avoided. Berries are low in sugar, especially blueberries, and can be added to juice recipes. Green apples (such as Granny Smith or Pippin) are lower in

> sugar than yellow or red apples. But I don't recommend that you use even green apples unless you are on your way to getting your blood sugar under control. Keep your juices and your entire diet very low in sugar.
>
> I've worked with people who have reversed their diabetes by juicing low-sugar vegetables and eating many more living foods, along with adopting a low-glycemic, high-fiber diet.

Vegetable juice promotes weight loss.

Two university studies have shown that one to two glasses of vegetable juice a day promote four times the weight loss of non-juice drinkers on the same American Heart Association diet. Both studies were randomized controlled trials, each lasting twelve week.[11]

In the study conducted by University of California–Davis among ninety healthy adults between the ages of forty and sixty-five, it was found that each person who drank at least two cups of vegetable juice a day met their weight-loss goal while only 7 percent of the non-juice drinkers met it. Participants who drank either one or two cups of vegetable juice per day lost an average of four pounds, while those who drank no vegetable juice lost only one pound. The researchers also found that people in the vegetable-juice groups had significantly higher vitamin C and potassium intake and a significantly lower intake of carbohydrates.[12] Participants with borderline high blood pressure who drank one or two cups of vegetable juice lowered their blood pressure significantly.[13]

The vegetable juice drinkers said they enjoyed the juice and felt as if they were doing something good for themselves by drinking it. According to Carl Keen, PhD, professor of Nutrition and Internal Medicine at University of California–Davis and coauthor of the study, "Enjoyment is so critical to developing good eating habits you can stick with for the long-term.... Vegetable juice is something that people enjoy, plus it's convenient and portable, which makes it simple to drink every day."[14]

A Baylor College of Medicine study involved eighty-one adults who drank eight to sixteen ounces of vegetable juice daily as part of a calorie-controlled, heart-healthy diet. They showed an average of four pounds lost during a twelve-week study period compared with those who did not drink juice and lost only one pound. Of the participants in the study—almost three-quarters of whom were women—83 percent had metabolic syndrome, which is a cluster of risk factors, including excess body fat around the midsection, high blood pressure, high blood sugar, insulin resistance, low HDL, and elevated triglycerides and cholesterol.[15] It is estimated that 47 million Americans have some combination of these risk factors. If not corrected by following a low-glycemic diet, this syndrome usually evolves into diabetes.[16] Most of the people with metabolic syndrome in the study lost weight when adding vegetable juice to their diet, four times the weight of others who did not drink juice.

NEGATIVE CALORIE JUICING

Drink a glass of vegetable juice before each meal to help curb you appetite. If you choose the ingredients with care, you can get a double dividend of appetite control. The best vegetables to use when juicing for weight loss are *negative calorie foods*—those that require more calories to digest than they contain. Choose foods such as dark greens, broccoli, carrots, Jerusalem artichoke, fennel, and cabbage. Also consider using asparagus, cucumber, and celery, which are natural diuretics that can alleviate water retention.

Vegetable juice stabilizes blood sugar.

Because it's very low in sugar, vegetable juice can also play an important role in stabilizing blood sugar, a vital factor in appetite control. Now that's something to get excited about! Sugar and refined flour products (such as bread, rolls, and pasta) that quickly turn into sugar in your body cause spikes and dips in blood sugar. When your blood sugar gets low, you can get ravenously hungry and sometimes grouchy. The sugar percentage of vegetable juice is much lower than that of fruit juice and the calorie count is up to 50 percent less, yet the juice succeeds in satisfying a sweet tooth. Amazing! This make juicing an absolute must for successful dieting. Experiment with greens such as kale, chard, or collard combined with lemon and ginger; or try a combination of carrot, Jerusalem artichoke (also known as sun choke), lemon, and parsley juice when a carb craving hits. The juice jolt will give those cravings a knockout!

SPRINKLE CINNAMON IN YOUR JUICE

Researchers have suggested that people with diabetes may see improvements by adding ¼ to 1 teaspoon of cinnamon to their food. A twelve-week London study involved fifty-eight type 2 diabetics. After twelve weeks on 2 grams (about ½ teaspoon) of cinnamon per day, study subjects had significantly lowered blood-sugar levels, as well as significantly reduced blood pressures.[17] Experts recommend Ceylon cinnamon over the more common cassia cinnamon because it contains significantly higher levels of cinnamon oil compared to cassia varieties and upwards of two hundred times more coumarin. It is more expensive but well worth it.

When you satisfy your body with nutrient-dense juices and foods and your blood sugar stabilizes, you appetite for junk food, sweets, and high-carb fare begins to fade away. You may notice your fatigue vanishing and your energy zooming. You will feel more like getting up and going in the morning, working out, and getting things done. Like so many other juicing enthusiasts, you may also notice that your focus improves dramatically. That's because your brain is being well fed. When you eat nutrient-depleted food, your brain doesn't get as many of the raw materials it needs to make reactions happen. Things misfire, and you walk around looking for your car keys for ten minutes when they're in your pocket the whole time. Now you can say good-bye to brain fog!

SUCCESS STORY

I was diagnosed with diabetes about a two months ago. I really didn't like taking the medication because of the side effects. My goal was to heal my body with good nutrition so I wouldn't need medication any longer. To achieve my goal, I stopped consuming so many dairy products, which are high in sugar. Instead of milk, I began drinking freshly made vegetable juices. I lowered my carbohydrate intake as well. In 30 days I lost 20 pounds! I cut my medication in half because my blood sugar fell too low. I was very encouraged by how quickly my body responded to my dietary changes. My goal is to get off the medication completely and control my blood sugar with good diet choices.

—Fr. Gregory

Roadblocks to Diabetic Weight Loss

Insulin resistance, metabolic syndrome, and insufficient sleep are all factors that can impede weight loss.

Insulin resistance

Insulin resistance causes weight gain because it disrupts fat metabolism. When the cells won't absorb the extra glucose circulating in the bloodstream, the liver converts it into fat. And guess what? Normal fat cells are loaded with glucose receptors that are sensitive to insulin signals. So while the fat cells are gobbling up glucose, the other cells are actually "starved" for glucose. A person with this condition feels tired a lot and tends to eat more carbohydrate-rich foods, trying to boost energy, which makes the situation even worse. It becomes a frustrating cycle.

A healthy body is insulin sensitive, not insulin resistant. Today most of the calories in an average American diet come from carbohydrates, with many of those being simple carbohydrates—sugars in the form of sweets and refined flour—that quickly enter the bloodstream. The body has to release high levels of insulin to keep the level of glucose in the bloodstream from spiraling out of control.

Letting your blood sugar get too high is simply not acceptable to your body. The resulting excess of insulin in your bloodstream is called hyperinsulinemia. Your body wasn't designed for prolonged high levels of insulin; it disrupts cellular metabolism and spreads inflammation. Over time the cells quit responding to this signal, and the body becomes insulin resistant. It's like knocking on a person's door to the point of annoyance; no one answers.

Metabolic syndrome

Although Gerald Reaven, MD, professor emeritus at Stanford School of Medicine, first identified metabolic syndrome in 1998, its principal component of obesity was not initially emphasized. Metabolic syndrome is a combination of obesity, hypercholesterolemia, and hypertension linked by an underlying insulin resistance. Any three of the following traits in an individual signify metabolic syndrome:

- Abdominal obesity: a waist circumference over 102 centimeters (40 inches) in men and over 88 centimeters (35 inches) in women

- High serum triglycerides: 150 mg/dl or above

- Low HDL cholesterol: 40 mg/dl or lower in men and 50 mg/dl or lower in women

- High blood pressure: 130/85 or more

- High blood sugar: a fasting blood glucose of 110 mg/dl or above (some groups say 100 mg/dl)

Metabolic syndrome is also associated with excess insulin secretion. Normally the body monitors the food we've digested, our blood-sugar levels, and our cell demands and releases insulin in the right amounts for our needs. The insulin then signals the cells to absorb glucose from the bloodstream. But excessive dietary intake of sugar and refined flour products, lack of exercise, and genetic tendencies contribute to insulin resistance and the other characteristics that lead to metabolic syndrome.

The lifestyle changes that turn this syndrome around start with a low-glycemic diet and avoidance of *all* sugar.

Eliminate sugar and reduce fruit. As mentioned earlier, juice only low-sugar fruit such as green apple or berries, lemon and lime. Sweeteners, no matter what we call them, are still sugars. Most natural sweeteners such as honey, brown rice syrup, and pure maple syrup are a little better than refined sugars in that they have some nutrients and aren't bleached and refined; however, they are still sugar.

The one sweetener you can use in small amounts is stevia. But we aware that a lot of stevia today has other sugar added to it. Don't be fooled. Get only pure stevia. I recommend Sweet Leaf Vanilla Creme, our favorite in the Calbom house.

In addition, avoid caffeine and tobacco. Include plenty of healthy fats, especially the omega-3 fats, and avoid animal fats. Limit your salt intake, and make sure you exercise at least three to four times per week. All this should help your cells become more responsive to insulin and curb overproduction of insulin. Weight loss should follow without a lot of effort. But the best news is that your health will improve immensely.

Insufficient sleep

In our frenzy to get everything done, we're missing out on one of our body's most important needs—a good night's sleep. A whopping one-third of our population sleeps only six and a half hours or less nightly—far less than the eight hours many sleep specialists recommend.

Research is showing that there is a correlation between the lack of sleep so many Americans are experiencing and the weight gain that is plaguing our nation. "We've known that people use food as a pick-me-up when they are tired, but now it appears they are hungrier than we realized, and there is a hormonal basis for their eating," says Thomas Wadden, director of the Weight and Eating Disorders Program at the University of Pennsylvania in Philadelphia.[18]

Columbia University studied the sleep habits of 3,682 people and found that those who got by on less than four hours of sleep a night were 73 percent more likely to be obese than those who slept seven to nine hours nightly. Those catching a moderate six hours of sleep a night were 23 percent more likely to be obese.[19]

If you've thought sleeping was a waste of time, you don't need to feel guilty about sleeping ever again. There are hormones that make you hungry and hormones that control your appetite. Research shows they are significantly influenced by how much sleep you get. Here's what studies have revealed:

- Five major appetite-influencing hormones can get out of whack when you don't get enough sleep, which significantly affects how much food you eat.[20] When you are sleep-deprived, your metabolism can really suffer, which causes weight gain.[21]

- Appetite-suppressing hormones and appetite-stimulating hormones are best regulated when you get seven to nine hours of sleep per night.[22]

- You won't tend to crave high-calorie, carbohydrate-rich foods nearly as much when you get adequate, refreshing sleep.[23]

- Sufficient sleep will help you manage your blood sugar more effectively, which helps you manage your appetite. Even one week of sleep deprivation can set off a temporary diabetic effect, causing you to crave sugar and other fattening foods.[24]

Over a period of years poor sleep patterns, along with poor eating habits and/or chronic stress, can also cause adrenal fatigue to develop. For example, someone who eats a lot of refined foods and sugar will have not only an imbalance in the hormone insulin but also in the hormone cortisol. Just as eating poorly over a long period of time can lead to insulin resistance and eventually diabetes, so also the constant secretion of cortisol in response to eating poorly and/or dealing with chronic stress can weaken the adrenal glands and eventually lead to adrenal fatigue.

Similarly not getting enough sleep can weaken the adrenals. Many people stay up late watching television, surfing the Internet, staying out with friends, or studying. They get too little sleep on a regular basis. An occasional short night of sleep is not a problem, but on a regular basis it can cause big health ramifications.

Rejoice! Sleeping in a few extra minutes has its advantages. Research shows that if you increase your sleep by just thirty minutes per night, your chances of losing weight go up exponentially.[25]

It's apparent that getting plenty of refreshing sleep on a consistent basis and enough sleep to meet your body's needs can be far better for your weight-loss goals than diet pills—and just as important as working out or eating right.

Chapter 4

DITCH THE SUGAR

FOR AT LEAST the past four decades Americans have shunned fats and gorged on sugar, which is a leading contributor to type 2 diabetes, metabolic syndrome, and excessive weight gain, as well as other diseases. It is true to say that nearly every disease—not only diabetes—has a link to sugar.[1]

Sugar in the amount that the typical American eats (about sixty-four pounds a year) continually upsets body chemistry and causes the inflammatory process that leads to disease. The less sugar you eat, the less inflammation and the stronger your immune system, which defends you against infectious and degenerative diseases. Excess sugar in the blood causes glycation, a process whereby a sugar molecule binds to a protein or a fat and leads to the formation of advanced glycation end products (AGEs). AGEs are inflammatory; they are associated with type 2 diabetes, aging, and many diseases.

Don't be fooled. Sugar is hidden in packaging in many different forms: high-fructose corn syrup, corn syrup solids, sucrose, maltose, dextrose, fructose, glucose, galactose, lactose. Most of it is found in sodas and other drinks, desserts, boxed cereals, energy bars, packaged snacks, premade foods, and flavored yogurt. In the United States much of the sugar added to foods is high-fructose corn syrup, which is used to sweeten everything from crackers to tomato sauce to ketchup to sodas to processed meats—and even some health-food products. It's used primarily because it's cheap.

43

When a manufacturer wants to sweeten a certain brand of cereal, for example, it can do this using either 15 grams of sugar or a combination of 5 grams of malt syrup, 5 grams of invert sugar, and 5 grams of glucose. Some manufacturers seem to be choosing this divide-and-masquerade method, placing these ingredients lower down on their products' lists to make the public believe that the amount of sugar in the product is smaller than it is.

Still, no matter the name, it is all sugar: evaporated cane juice, cane-juice solids, cane juice crystals, Sucanat, dextrin (a complex sugar molecule left over from enzyme action on starch), malto-dextrin, dextran, barley malt, beet sugar, caramel, buttered syrup, carob syrup, brown sugar (white sugar with molasses added), date sugar, malt syrup, diatastic malt (enzymes that break down starch into sugar), fruit juice concentrate, dehydrated fruit juice, fruit juice crystals, golden syrup, turbinado, sorghum syrup, molasses, refiner's syrup, maltitol, maple syrup, yellow rock sugar, xylitol (usually made from by-products of the wood-pulp industry or from cane pulp, seed hulls, or corn husks), and sugar alcohols such as sorbitol and mannitol.

People with diabetes need this information—and they also need to know where to turn when that freshly made glass of juice is just too tart to swallow. Here are some healthy alternative sweeteners (to be used in limited amounts, of course):

- Stevia (I recommend Sweet Leaf Vanilla Creme)
- Coconut sugar and coconut nectar
- Xylitol made from birch bark (avoid xylitol made from the pulp industry by-products)
- Small amounts of pure maple syrup
- Small amounts of local raw honey

HIGH-FRUCTOSE CORN SYRUP MAKES YOUR BRAIN CRAVE FOOD

The average American now consumes 145 pounds of high-fructose corn syrup per year. It's amazing we're not all obese and diabetic! New research proves exactly how high-fructose corn syrup bypasses normal energy balance systems in the body, causing the brain to want more food because it never really registers the calories of the high-fructose corn syrup.[2] There is also research indicating that high-fructose corn syrup turns on gene signaling that promotes fat formation and fat accumulation, which is likely to result in obesity, insulin resistance, and type 2 diabetes.[3]

What About Artificial Sweeteners?

People with diabetes often think that they can satisfy their sweet tooth safely with artificial sweeteners, but it's not a good idea. For the sake of your health—not just your weight— completely avoid all artificial sweeteners, which can cause a host of health problems. And if you think they're helping you lose weight, take a look at the research. People on sugar substitutes actually gain more weight than those using sugar.[4] Using either one—sugar or sugar substitutes—remains a very bad choice for your weight as well as for your health.

According to the late Dr. H. J. Roberts, the worst of the artificial sweetener lot is aspartame (brand name, NutraSweet). Dr. Roberts waged a decades-long campaign against the use of aspartame in products such as flavored waters, sodas, powdered drink mixes, cooking sauces, children's medicine, chewing gums, table sweeteners, and other "sugar-free" products, citing specific risks to pregnant and nursing mothers and their children. He calls the result of such use "aspartame disease" and warned in particular of its manifestations in young children, which include: severe headaches, convulsions, unexplained visual loss, rashes, asthma, gastrointestinal problems, obesity, marked weight loss, hypoglycemia, diabetes, addiction (probably largely due to the methyl alcohol), hyperthyroidism, and a host of neuropsychiatric features. The latter include extreme fatigue, irritability, hyperactivity, depression, antisocial behavior (including suicide), poor school performance, the deterioration of intelligence, and brain tumors. These manifestations tend to be magnified in patients with unrecognized hypothyroidism (underactive thyroid), hypoglycemia (low-blood-sugar reactions), diabetes, and phenylketonuria (PKU).[5]

Since a diagnosis of diabetes or prediabetes makes your health a primary concern, why compromise it further by substituting artificial sweeteners for other sugars? Believe me and many others who have successfully reduced the demands of their sweet tooth simply by deciding not to supply it with sweets anymore. You *can* retrain your taste buds, believe it or not!

Recommended Fruits

The sweetness of fruit is a different matter—within the guidelines of the glycemic index. You will remember from the previous chapter that a number of fruits, which are often preferred for juicing, are welcome (to a degree) in your diabetes menu plan.

Juicing does tend to concentrate many ingredients, however, since you may need to use more than a typical raw serving to get the desired flavor and volume. Therefore, especially until you have your blood sugar under control, I recommend that you stick with the lowest-sugar fruits—lemons, limes, and cranberries. Berries are also lower in sugar than many other fruits, so blueberries, strawberries, raspberries, blackberries, and more may be used. As you will see in the recipes later in this book, one technique for diluting a higher-sugar fruit in juicing is to add cucumber juice or dark leafy greens.

You can add cranberries to many recipes for a delicious enhancer to your juice drinks and a boost to your weight loss at the same time. If you buy these berries when they're in season, you can freeze a few packages to have on hand for seasons when they aren't available.

An added bonus regarding blueberries is that they can help you get rid of belly fat, thanks to the high level of phytochemicals (antioxidants) they contain. A study found that blueberries are helpful in preventing type 2 diabetes and that the benefits are even greater when the blueberries are combined with a low-fat diet.[6] Moreover, blueberries can also help fight hardening of the arteries and improve memory. Make sure you purchase only organic blueberries since their skin can carry unwelcome pesticide residues otherwise.

Lemons are wonderful. Adding just a tablespoon of freshly squeezed lemon juice to your glass of water, your salad, or your soup not only will make everything taste better but also will help ward off cravings and keep your insulin levels in check. Meyer lemons are my favorite because they are sweeter; they are available in the winter. Hot lemon water with a dash of cayenne is a great way to start your day—it gets the liver, your fat-burning organ, moving in the morning. It's also a natural diuretic and helps clear out toxins from your system. Further, it aids the digestive process and prevents constipation. It can also help alleviate heartburn—just add a tablespoon of fresh lemon juice to water and drink it with your meal. (Limonene, a compound in lemons, helps short-circuit the production of acid in your stomach—lemons are very alkalizing.)

SINGING THE BLUES

Food and mood are definitely connected. Sugar is one of the leading causes of "the blues." In 1975 William Dufty wrote the book *Sugar Blues*. What he said was right on target—and that was back when we didn't have sugar in just about everything we buy in a package. Recently I returned a package of sliced organic turkey to the store because, to my utter surprise, it contained sugar. It seems that ever since our nation went on a get-rid-of-all-fat craze, we've been dumping sugar into just about everything. The result is that depression is soaring, along with heart disease, cancer, and diabetes.

Low-Glycemic Juicing

The word "juice" refers to so much more than orange, grapefruit, or any other fruity, sweet juice on the breakfast menu. Some juices are green as grass. Some are hot and tongue-tingling. I love to explore new taste combinations and their health benefits! In this book you will discover recipe after recipe for delicious, satisfying juices that will make you forget you ever had a problem with your sweet tooth.

The goal for a person with diabetes is to juice fruits and vegetables that are low on the glycemic index. Low-glycemic foods, especially raw carbohydrates, can help control blood sugar, appetite, and weight. Though helpful for everyone, they are especially helpful for people with type 2 diabetes, prediabetes, hypoglycemia, insulin resistance, and metabolic syndrome. Low-glycemic foods are absorbed more slowly, allowing a person to feel full longer and therefore be less likely to overeat. Raw-food experts have found that raw carbohydrates such as raw juices are better

tolerated than cooked carbs. They don't elicit the addictive cravings that cooked foods cause. Experts believe that the enzymes in
raw food play an important role in the way they stimulate weight
loss, as they do in the treatment of obesity.[7]

The benefits of low-glycemic juicing are numerous. To review:
High-glycemic foods raise your blood-sugar levels, cause your
body to secrete excess insulin, and lead to the storage of fat. The
glycemic index helps diabetics manage blood sugar and works
well for weight loss as well.

Researchers reported in the *Journal of the American Medical
Association* that patients who lost weight with a low-glycemic diet
kept the weight off longer than patients who lost the same amount
of weight with a low-fat diet.[8] A GI diet ranks carbohydrates
according to how much a certain amount of each food raises a
person's blood sugar level. (Researchers figure out how much a
50-gram serving of carbohydrate raises a person's blood sugar
level compared with a control; see appendix B.) Virtually all carbohydrates are digested into glucose and cause a temporary rise
in blood-glucose levels; this is called the glycemic response. But
some foods elevate blood-glucose levels more than others. The glycemic response is affected by many factors, including the quantity
of food, the amount and type of carbohydrate, whether it's cooked
or eaten raw (and if cooked, how), and the degree of processing.
Each food is assigned an index number from 1 to 100, with 100
as the reference score for pure glucose. Typically foods are rated
high (greater than 70), moderate (56–69), and low (less than 55).
(See "Glycemic Index and Glycemic Load" in chapter 2.)

Detox Too

Remember that chemicals can interfere with your ability to
balance blood sugar and metabolize cholesterol and that, as time

goes on, these changes can lead to insulin resistance. "This scientific discovery should be headline news," says Dr. Mark Hyman, "but no one is talking about it because there are no drugs to treat it. In the quest to conquer the two biggest epidemics of our time—diabetes and obesity—we've got to turn our attention to the heavy burden environmental toxins put on our bodies."[9] Environmental toxins can contribute heavily (pun intended) to weight gain and also to diabetes.[10]

Dr. Hyman continues to discuss that if your body's detoxification system isn't working well, waste will build up. Over time the waste buildup is similar to what happens when trash collectors go on strike and don't pick up the garbage. The accumulated waste piles high, creating a breeding ground for illnesses. We live in a toxic environment; we are steeped in chemicals that our bodies are not designed to process. For a disturbing look at the chemicals that breach the boundaries of our bodies, look at the Centers for Disease Control and Prevention's National Report on Human Exposure to Environmental Chemicals. In a recent report scientists at the CDC found that nearly every person they tested was packing a host of nasty chemicals, including flame retardants stored in fatty tissue and bisphenol A (BPA), a hormonelike substance found in plastics. Even babies are contaminated.[11] In 2004 the Environmental Working Group tested the umbilical cord blood from ten newborns. The cord blood contained 287 chemicals—217 were neurotoxic (toxic to nerves or nervous tissue).[12]

Think about your body as you would your car. What if you never changed your oil or filters in your car? It's the same thing with your body. To keep it humming along like a well-maintained vehicle, you need to periodically cleanse the blood and its filter systems, which are your organs of elimination. If you are struggling to lose weight despite eating well and exercising, toxins may be interfering with your body's metabolism. There's a lot you can do when it comes to taking out your body's trash.

Because of all the environmental pollution in our world and our occasional, or maybe continual, unwise food choices, our normal body processes can get overwhelmed. Toxic substances, mucus, and congestion get trapped in our tissues and tissue spaces. Our body attempts to protect us by enclosing toxins in mucus and fat cells, and it will hang onto those fat cells to save us. We may not be able to lose weight unless we cleanse our bodies first. The same goes for getting well and achieving vibrant health.

It's estimated that the average adult has between five and ten pounds of accumulated toxic waste in their cells, tissues, and organs, particularly the colon. (That's five to ten pounds we could feel really great about dropping!) Toxic substances that accumulate throughout the body can weaken and congest our organs and systems of elimination and lead to diseases such as cancer. They also mess up our weight-loss goals. If we go on a very strict diet that forces the body to let go of fat cells for survival, the weight will come right back on when we stop the program.

Toxins come not only from the environment and unhealthy food choices but also from the internal by-products of metabolism called "endotoxins." The endotoxins in our bodies mix with the environmental toxins, and we have a conglomeration of nasty stuff swimming around inside us. This toxic soup mix consists of chemicals, pesticides, drug residues, heavy metals, and food additives, along with by-products from digestion as well as yeasts, fungus, and parasites. This stuff can pile up inside the body like gunk inside home plumbing. If it is not broken down and eliminated, it gets stored in the body. The body especially likes to store it in fat cells; it's one of the safest places to put them. It will even make more of these little storage units as needed.

This toxic stuff can also jam up the works in organs such as the liver and kidneys. It can be found in the large and the small intestines. And it hides in the mucous lining of the lungs and sinuses. It gets deposited in the skin and bones as well. Additionally toxins are distributed into the cells and tissues of the brain, where they can cause a lot of cognitive and emotional problems such as "brain fog" and emotional outbursts.

Toxins make us sick, weak, overweight, and unable to fight off infection, and they cause pain in our muscles and joints. Toxic molecules known as free radicals damage our cells, creating numerous health problems and accelerating aging. This is why it's so crucial to periodically cleanse the body.

HOW TOXIC ARE YOU?

Do you have symptoms of toxicity? Take the toxicity quiz below and give yourself a point for every symptom that describes you. But even if you don't score any points, you should detox your body at least once a year. It's like changing your vehicle's oil. You don't wait until your car starts having problems; you change the oil to keep the car "symptom free." As you cleanse each organ of elimination, you'll improve your health, become stronger, look younger, and remain symptom-free.

- Aches and pains
- Acid reflux
- Arthritis
- Bloating and gas
- Cellulite
- Constipation
- Dizziness

- Emotional and mental problems
- Headaches
- Hormone imbalances
- Inability to lose weight
- Indigestion
- Irritability
- Lack of energy and fatigue
- Overweight
- Premature aging
- Restlessness
- Sinus problems
- Skin problems
- Stressful feelings
- Trouble sleeping/insomnia
- Visual problems
- Weakness

Eliminating Toxins

Don't despair if you scored high on the toxicity quiz. Raw juices and live foods are chock-full of antioxidants, which bind to toxins and carry them out of the body. Antioxidants latch onto the "bad guys" just as Pac-Man in the video game eats every dot or power pellet.

To get rid of accumulating toxins, add specific cleanse programs to your healthy juicing and eating plan. You can read about these in detail in my book *Juicing, Fasting, and Detoxing for Life* and hear about them on my DVD, *Detoxing for Health*. I help you put the cleanses into practice with my 30-Day Detox Challenge online e-course. You can find out more about these detox products on my Juice Lady website.[13]

Fresh vegetable juices should be an integral part of your overall lifestyle regimen because they promote health in a variety of ways. The concentration of vitamins, minerals, phytoneutrients, biophotons, and enzymes that juicing provides gives the body extra stamina and boosts the immune system. My recommendation is that you drink two glasses of veggie juice each day. It's best to drink one glass in the morning and one in the afternoon or before dinner. If this schedule isn't possible, then drink the juices whenever you can. You can make them the night before and take the juice to work in a stainless steel water bottle or thermos. You can store them (covered) in the refrigerator for up to twenty-four hours without losing significant amounts of nutrients, although the longer it sits, the more nutrients it will lose. And if you are really busy, you can juice a big batch and freeze it in individual glass containers. (Tip: Don't fill the jars to the top or they'll burst when they freeze.)

Plain green tea (no sugar), white tea, or herbal teas are other great additions to your healthy lifestyle. But good old H_2O— purified, that is—is the best of all. A good water purifier is a great investment. (If you take the purified water with you to work or on the road, carry it in stainless steel or glass water bottles to avoid the plastic toxins that are leached into water from plastic bottles.)

For sparkling water, choose mineral water that is naturally carbonated such as S. Pellegrino or Apollinaris instead of commercially gassed varieties.

Whatever you choose to do, completely avoid soft drinks, because they are like drinking liquid candy with chemicals caustic enough to rust nails. Soft drinks are loaded with sugar or artificial sweeteners, and numerous studies have connected them with weight gain and other health problems. Along the same lines, watch out for sweetened bottled teas, energy drinks, sports drinks, and vitamin-infused water.

Sugar Is Not Your Friend

As you well know, in your lifelong fight against diabetes sugar is *not* your friend. However, you can't "unfriend" sugar in your life if you don't know where it is hiding. Learn how to read labels.

More important, learn which fresh foods are best for you. It may seem too complicated to learn about "glycemic load" and new ways of combining healthy foods into your diet with fresh juices, snacks, and meals, but it will be well worth it if you can get your blood sugar under control and keep it stabilized.

Denying the demands of your one little sweet tooth is not a high price to pay—after all, the health of your entire body is at stake.

EIGHT REASONS TO DITCH SUGAR

Here are a few *top tips* to motivate you to ditch the sugar in your diet.

- Sugar causes diabetes, kidney and heart problems. Excess sugar can damage the pancreas's ability to function properly.

- Sugar is a major contributor to inflammation. Inflammation is a top cause of heart disease and nearly all other diseases.

- Sugar makes you fat. It is loaded with calories that are stored in fat cells.

- Sugar is toxic.

- Sugar will raise your cholesterol. For years we were told it was fat that raised our cholesterol, but sugar is worse.

- Sugar makes you nervous. There is a clear link between excess sugar and disorders such as anxiety, depression, and schizophrenia because of the high levels of insulin and adrenalin that get released with sugar consumption.

- Sugar destroys your teeth. It increases the bacteria in your mouth that erodes enamel.

- Sugar suppresses the immune system. Sugar beats out vitamin C in your immune cells and weakens them.

- Sugar causes wrinkles. A high-sugar diet damages collagen, the layer just below the skin that gives you that youthful appearance.

Chapter 5

WHY JUICE?

O K, SO I'VE convinced you of the importance of losing weight, detoxing, and eliminating sugar from your diet as the means of improving your overall health and helping to manage your blood-sugar levels. "But why juice?" you may object. "Doesn't juice deliver its nutrition too fast for someone with sugar metabolism problems? I've been told that juice is one of the quickest ways to get a sugar spike."

Yes, you *can* juice—if you choose low-sugar veggies and fruits such as lemons and berries. The key to keeping your blood sugar balanced is to balance what you consume. Juicing is a wonderful way to get an amazing amount of nutrition in a tasty form, quickly. But it is important to combine it with a low-glycemic, high-fiber, often high-protein diet to help your system out and stabilize your blood sugar.

How many times have you eaten a meal and not long after, you felt tired, lethargic, or spacey? Obviously that food was not a good choice. Yet often we keep eating the same things over and over again, even though they don't help us feel better, more energized, or more alert. Eat foods that love you back. Fresh juices, especially fresh veggie juices, will love you back all the time by giving you energy, vitality, and better mental performance.

I hope to inspire you to make juicing a daily habit.

All About Juicing

I want to tell you more about juicing so that you can get started. First I'll explain the equipment you'll need. Then I'll tell you how to select your ingredients so that you can make the best juices in the world right in your own kitchen.

How to choose the right juicer

Choosing a juicer that is right for you can make the difference between juicing daily and never juicing again, so it's important to get one that works for your lifestyle.

People often ask me if they can use their blender as a juicer. My answer: *You can't use a blender to make juice no matter how high-powered or expensive it is.* A juicer separates the liquid from the pulp (insoluble fiber). A blender liquefies everything that is placed in it; it doesn't separate the insoluble fiber from the juice. If you think it might be a good idea to have carrot, beet, parsley, and celery pulp in your juice for added fiber, I can tell you from experience that it tastes like juicy mush.

For the best juice, which is juice you'll enjoy and drink every day, you need a juicer. Which one is the best? The one you will use all the time! Look for the following features:

- *Adequate horsepower (hp).* I recommend a juicer with 0.3 to 0.5 hp. Weak-motored machines with low horsepower ratings must run at extremely high rpm (revolutions per minute). A machine's rpm does not accurately reflect its ability to perform effectively because rpm is calculated when the juicer is running idle, not while it is juicing. When you feed produce into a low-power machine, the rpm will be reduced dramatically, and sometimes the juicer will come to a full stop. I have "killed" some machines on the first celery rib I juiced.

- *Efficient at extracting juice.* I've used a number of juicers that wasted a lot of produce because there was a lot of juice left in the pulp. You should not be able to squeeze a lot of juice out of the pulp. Some machines' rpm is too high and the pulp comes out very wet. You can waste a lot of money on produce because of an inefficient juicer.

- *Sustains blade speed during juicing.* Look for a machine that has electronic circuitry that sustains blade speed during juicing.

- *Able to juice all types of produce.* Make sure the machine can juice tough, hard vegetables as well as delicate greens. Make sure it doesn't need a special citrus attachment. For wheatgrass juice (more on that later), you'll need a wheatgrass juicer or a juicer that presses the juice, such as a single-auger or twin-gear machine, also known as a masticating juicer. Be aware that the machines that juice wheatgrass along with other vegetables and fruit take more time to use. Some are more time-consuming to clean as well.

- *Large feed tube.* Look for a large feed tube if you don't have a lot of time to devote to juicing. Cutting your produce into small pieces before juicing does take time. The masticating-style juicers have small openings at the top.

- *Ejects pulp.* Choose a juicer that ejects pulp into a receptacle. This design is far better than one in which all the pulp stays inside the machine and has to be scooped out frequently. Juicers that keep the pulp in the center basket rather than ejecting it cannot juice continuously. You'll need to stop the machine often to wash it out. Plus, you can line the pulp catcher with a free plastic baggie from the grocery store produce section and you won't have to wash the receptacle each time. When you're done juicing, you can either toss the pulp or use it in cooking or composting.

- *Easy to clean.* Look for a juicer with only a few parts to clean. The more parts a juicer has, and the more complicated the parts are to wash, the longer it will take to clean up, and the more time it will take to put it back together. That makes it less likely you will use your machine daily. Also, make sure the parts are dishwasher safe. It's very easy to just rinse the parts and let them air dry. For the blade basket, it really helps to spray it, if you have a separate faucet sprayer. This can blow out fiber particles very quickly. Then take a soft-bristle dish brush and brush both sides quickly under running water. I clean the lid, blade basket, and juice bowl in this manner in less than a minute.

Juicing guidelines

Juicing is a very simple process. Even if you're not much of a cook, you can do it. Simple as the procedure is, though, it helps to keep a few guidelines in mind to get the best results.

- *Wash all produce before juicing.* Fruit and vegetable washes are available at many grocery and health food stores. Or you can use hydrogen peroxide and then rinse. Cut away all moldy, bruised, or damaged areas of the produce.

- *Always peel oranges, tangerines, tangelos, and grapefruit before juicing.* The skins of these citrus fruits contain volatile oils that can cause digestive problems such as stomachaches. Lemon and lime peels can be juiced, if organic, but they do add a distinct flavor that is not one of my favorites for most recipes. I usually peel them. Leave as much of the white pithy part on the citrus fruit as possible, though, since it contains the most vitamin C and bioflavonoids. Bioflavonoids work with vitamin C; they need each other to create the best uptake for your immune cells. If you use mangoes, always peel them, since their skins contain an irritant that is harmful when eaten in quantity.

- *Peel all produce that is not labeled organic* even though the largest concentration of nutrients is in and next to the skin. For example, nonorganic cucumbers are often waxed, trapping the pesticides. You don't want the wax or pesticides in your juice. The peels and skins of sprayed fruits and vegetables contain the largest concentration of pesticides.

- *Remove pits, stones, and hard seeds* from fruits such as peaches, plums, apricots, cherries, and mangoes. Softer seeds from cucumbers, oranges, lemons, limes, watermelons, cantaloupes, and apples can be juiced without a problem. Because of their chemical composition, large quantities of apple seeds should not be juiced for young children under the age of two but should not cause problems for older children and adults.

- *Safely juice the stems and leaves of most produce* such as beet stems and leaves, strawberry caps, and

celery leaves; they offer nutrients too. But don't juice
carrot tops or rhubarb greens because they contain
toxic substances. Many recipes specify wrapping some
of the produce in the larger leaves of greens such as
lettuce for easier insertion into the juicer.

- *Cut fruits and vegetables into sections or chunks
  that will fit your juicer's feed tube.* You'll learn from
  experience what can be added whole and what size
  works best for your machine. If you have a large feed
  tube, you won't have to cut up a lot of produce.

- *Be aware that some fruits and vegetables don't juice
  well.* Most produce contains a lot of water, which
  makes it ideal for juicing. Vegetables and fruits that
  contain less water, such as avocados, will not juice
  as well. But they can be used in smoothies and cold
  soups by first juicing other produce, then pouring
  the juice into a blender, and adding the avocado, for
  example, to make a raw soup. Mangoes will juice but
  will make a thicker juice.

- *Drink your juice as soon as you can after it's made
  to get the most nutrients.*

- *Make juice ahead of time if necessary.* If you can't
  drink the juice right away, store it in an insulated container such as a thermos or another airtight, opaque
  container, and in the refrigerator if possible. You can
  store for up to twenty-four hours. Light, heat, and air
  will destroy nutrients quickly. Be aware that the longer
  juice sits before you drink it, the more nutrients are
  lost. If juice turns brown, it has oxidized and lost a
  large amount of its nutritional value; it is not good to

drink it as it may be spoiled. Melon and cabbage juice
do not store well; drink them soon after juicing.

- *Freeze juice you make in advance.* Not everyone can
  make juice each day. So make it when you can. Maybe
  that's the weekend. You can freeze the juice in individual containers such as glass jars. Make sure you
  don't fill them all the way to the top, however, because
  they will expand and burst.

What about fiber?

You may be wondering, "Don't we need the fiber that's lost
in juicing?" It's true that we need to eat whole vegetables, fruit,
sprouts, legumes, and whole grains for their fiber. Whole fruits
and vegetables have insoluble and soluble fiber. Both types of
fiber are very important to include in your diet. It's true that the
insoluble fiber is lost when you juice. However, soluble fiber is
present in juice in the form of gums and pectins. Soluble fiber is
excellent for the digestive tract. It also helps to lower blood cholesterol, stabilize blood sugar, and improve good bowel bacteria.

Don't worry about the fiber that is lost when you juice. Think
about all the extra nutrition you are getting. Fresh juice is one
of the best vitamin-mineral cocktails you could drink. You may
not need as many nutritional supplements when you juice, so that
could save you money in the long run. Drink your juice as a smart
addition to your high-fiber diet.

Although people used to think that a lot of nutrients got lost
with the fiber after juicing (because they remained with the
fiber), that theory has been disproved. The U.S. Department of
Agriculture analyzed twelve fruits and found that 90 percent of
the antioxidant nutrients they measured could be found in the

juice rather than the fiber.[1] This makes fresh juice a great supplement in the diet.

How much produce do I need?

People often ask me if it takes a bushel basket of produce to make a glass of juice. Actually, if you're using a good juicer, it takes a surprisingly small amount. For example, one large cucumber yields an eight-ounce glass of juice. The following each yield about four ounces of juice: one large apple, three to four large (thirteen-inch) ribs of celery, or one large orange. The key is to get a good juicer that yields a dry pulp. I've used juicers that ejected very wet pulp. When I ran the pulp through the juicer again I got more juice and the pulp was still wet. If the rpm is too high or the juicer is not efficient in other ways, you will waste a lot of produce.

What about the cost? Depending on your area of the country and availability, you will probably spend $2.00 to $3.50 per glass of juice, which might sound steep until you recognize the hidden savings. (But making juice yourself is also a true bargain compared to many juice bars, where you will pay $6.00 to $9.00 for a glass of juice.) First of all, no one can efficiently chew up the large amounts of veggies that go into a typical glass of juice—trust me, I have tried! But just think—you may not need as many vitamin supplements or over-the-counter medications such as painkillers, sleeping aids, antacids, and cold, cough, and flu medications. You may never run out of sick days again. With the immune-building, disease-fighting properties of fresh juice, you should stay well all year long.

WASTE NOT, WANT NOT

Start saving parts of vegetables to juice that you would normally toss such as the stems of broccoli, the base of cauliflower, the tough stems of asparagus, radish leaves, kohlrabi leaves, cilantro stems, parsley stems, spinach stems, kale ribs, and any other judicable part you may otherwise overlook. Add these parts to various juice recipes. If you add them in limited quantities, you won't even know they are there. This is great economy and good for your health.

Save your veggie pulp and add it to soups. (Use no more than two cups per soup recipe.) Try some of the dessert recipes in *The Juice Lady's Sugar Knockout* such as the Beet Brownies (using beet pulp) or the Chocolate Peanut Pulp Balls (using carrot pulp). Or save veggie pulp to feed your chickens. (It gives their eggs bright yellow yolks.) You can also compost it for rich garden soil.

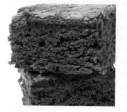

The Power of Green Juice

In addition to some of the basic steps described in chapter 3 that you can take to achieve weight-loss success, there are specific foods you can add to your weight-loss program that will make a huge difference in assisting your body to burn fat. These super-foods can help you succeed and give you super-size health dividends at the same time. *First on the list is green juice: the number-one fat cure.*

In honor of his hundredth show Dr. Oz served on the set his favorite green juice drink to one hundred people who had lost thirteen thousand pounds combined. This blend of cucumbers, apple, and leafy greens started a new wave of interest in green juices for weight loss. So why do green juices work so well? Dr. Oz claims that they compensate for the fact that most of us are simply not getting sufficient nourishment from standard diets. He says, "We know we have to have at least five fistfuls of leafy green vegetables and fruit every day, so we make a morning green drink."[2]

There's evidence to suggest that even if we took the time to chew up five cups of green veggies each day, we wouldn't get as much benefit from them as we would from juicing them. The mechanical process of juicing the vegetables breaks apart plant cell walls and makes absorption better than when food is chewed by even the most conscientious chewers—at least thirty times before swallowing. Juicing has an effect like that of throwing marbles rather than tennis balls at a chain-link fence; the juiced fruits and vegetables go through the digestive system in a way that "tennis balls" (larger bits of food) cannot.

The best news is that juices contain easily absorbed micronutrients that will do *more* than slim you down—they'll optimize your overall health and wellness. How? There's science behind the green juices' transformative powers that explains why juices help energize your body, fire up your metabolism, speed slimming, and overhaul your health. It is based on the activity of the nutrients they contain.

Magnesium

Magnesium-rich greens ramp up your energy. A British study comparing the metabolism of female twins found that magnesium intake was the most important dietary variable that determined adiponectin levels.[3] Adiponectin is a fat-cell hormone that promotes insulin sensitivity. This hormone has recently gained attention from researchers because of its regulation of glucose and fat metabolism. Elevated levels of adiponectin are associated with increased insulin sensitivity and fat burning. Adiponectin also seems to work closely with leptin—a hormone that helps control the appetite and boosts metabolism. As you lose weight with green juices, this hormone, which is made in the fat cells, gets a boost because fresh fruit and vegetables have a positive influence on it. Adiponectin also helps regulate inflammation, which, consequently, helps to prevent you from gaining weight, becoming a type 2 diabetic, or developing heart disease.

A person's nutritional intake must include adequate magnesium in order to maintain adiponectin levels. This points to a deficiency of magnesium (which is common in America), as a clear contributor to the problems people have with weight management. Magnesium also plays a key role in fighting off stress and anxiety, supporting restful sleep, preventing restless leg syndrome, and boosting energy.

Further, magnesium helps prevent fat storage. When magnesium is low, cells fail to recognize insulin. As a result, glucose accumulates in the blood—and then it gets stored as fat instead of being burned for fuel.

Green plants, which are rich in magnesium, are far superior to magnesium supplements because the supplements' particles are a bit large for the body to entirely absorb. (I'm in favor of taking magnesium supplements, if they are needed, but as an adjunct to a magnesium-rich diet.) Green plants take inorganic minerals from the soil through their tiny roots and incorporate them into their cells. They become organic particles that are much smaller and easier for the body to absorb. It is estimated that more than 90 percent of a plant's minerals is delivered to the cells when you juice the greens. So juice up those leaves—chard, collard, beet tops, parsley, spinach—the five highest in magnesium, plus kohlrabi leaves, kale, dandelion greens, dark green lettuce, and mustard greens.

MAGNESIUM-RICH GREENS

- Chard
- Collard
- Beet tops
- Parsley
- Spinach
- Kohlrabi leaves
- Kale
- Dandelion greens
- Lettuce (dark green)
- Mustard greens

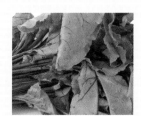

Vitamin K

Further, the high level of vitamin K in greens helps to promote the production of osteocalcin, a hormone that anchors calcium inside the bone and increases both insulin secretion and sensitivity. It also boosts the number of insulin-producing cells while reducing stores of fat. One study found that the risk of hip fracture in middle-aged women was reduced significantly by consuming vitamin K-rich vegetables. The *American Journal of Clinical Nutrition* reported, "Women who consumed lettuce one or more times per day had a significant 45% lower risk of hip fracture than women who consumed lettuce one or fewer times per week."[4]

Beta-carotene

Green leafy vegetables are also rich in beta-carotene, which can be converted to vitamin A in the body as it is needed. Greens contain nutrients that help immune function. And green vegetables are a very good source of iron and calcium. However, Swiss chard, beet greens, and spinach are not considered good sources of calcium due to their high content of oxalic acid, a natural compound that interferes with the absorption of calcium. This does not mean that you should avoid eating them because they are rich in many nutrients such as chlorophyll, magnesium, and vitamin K, but rather include them with other greens that are rich in absorbable calcium such as collards, kale, turnip greens, parsley, and watercress.

Sulforaphane

Sulforaphane is a compound in broccoli that can help reverse the damage that diabetes inflicts on blood vessels. It encourages the production of enzymes that protect the blood vessels and reduces the number of molecules that cause cell damage, known as reactive oxygen species (ROS), by up to 73 percent.

You can juice all parts of the broccoli, including the stems; you can add them to most recipes and reap the rewards. This is good economy and adds great nutrition.

Other nutrients

Dark-green leafy vegetables are rich in lutein, zeaxanthin, and other carotenoids needed in the lens of the eye and macular region of the retina. They help protect the eyes against both cataracts and macular degeneration, two major causes of blindness in older people. Lutein and zeaxanthin also reduce the risk of certain types of cancer such as breast and lung cancer. And they may also contribute to the prevention of heart disease and stroke.

In short, greens offer the nectar of life. Include them often in your juice recipes. They'll love you back every time! There are so many leafy greens to choose—collard, Swiss chard, curly kale, black dino kale, spinach, lettuces such as romaine and green leaf, watercress, parsley, beet greens, dandelion greens, and kohlrabi leaves. These vegetables are among the healthiest choices you can make for juicing.

GREEN VEGGIES HELP LOWER THE RISK OF TYPE 2 DIABETES

Because of their high magnesium content and low glycemic index, green leafy vegetables are also valuable for persons with type 2 diabetes. One study revealed that an increase of just one and one half servings a day of green leafy vegetables was associated with a 14 percent lower risk of diabetes.[5]

As we have seen, green juice has many benefits for your body. Besides helping you lose weight, it will increase your energy and improve your overall health. That means you'll get more done and feel more like working out, so you'll burn even more calories and build more muscle.

Remember, the sooner you drink fresh juice after you make it, the more nutrients you'll get. However, you can store juice and not lose too many nutrients by keeping it cold, such as in an insulated container or in a covered container in the refrigerator. You can also freeze it.

BOOST YOUR METABOLISM

To boost your metabolism more than you can with green veggies alone, look for ways to include these three ingredients in your juices.

- *Apple cider vinegar:* A 2009 study shows that vinegar reduces body weight, body fat mass, and serum triglyceride levels. Turns out that apple cider vinegar can help your body burn 3.7 pounds over a 12-week period.[6]

- *Cinnamon:* Helps to regulate blood-sugar levels so excess fat does not build up. It helps accomplish this by controlling insulin levels.

- *Cayenne:* Revs up your metabolism. The component that does the work is capsaicin, which raises your body temperature and causes a boost in metabolism.

Here is a recipe that uses all three:

Spicy Apple Cider Vinegar Elixir[7]

24 oz. purified water
¼ cup of apple cider vinegar
½ tsp. of cayenne
1 tsp. of cinnamon
1 tsp. of raw honey
Juice of half a lemon

Mix all ingredients in a shaker jar or blender on low speed.

Wheatgrass

What about wheatgrass? It's often the first thing you think of when someone says "green juice." Wheatgrass (scientific name: *Triticum aestivum*) is an herb from the wheat family.[8] Usually consumed raw (juiced, below), wheatgrass is an excellent source of many vitamins and minerals, including vitamins A, C, E, K, B-complex, iron, calcium, magnesium, selenium, amino acids, and chlorophyll.[9]

According to the article on the Livestrong website titled "The Benefits of Wheatgrass for Diabetes":

> Wheatgrass has a definite role in improving glucose and lipids levels and can effectively be used in the management of diabetes, suggests a research team in a study published in the December 2099 issue of the *Journal of Herbal Medicine and Toxicology*....The researchers found that adding 15 grams of wheatgrass to certain foods significantly lowered the GI [glycemic index] of those foods and thus improved blood glucose levels. The blood levels of some fats called triglycerides were also improved in the participants who consumed wheatgrass.[10]

You can purchase ready-made wheatgrass juice or wheatgrass powder, or you can acquire freshly harvested wheatgrass at a health food store or grocery store and make your own. You can also grow your own wheatgrass. Freshly cut wheatgrass should keep fresh for about a week in the refrigerator.

In order to juice wheatgrass, you'll need a wheatgrass juicer or a juicer that presses the juice, such as a single-auger or twin-gear machine—also known as a masticating juicer. Plan ahead: juicing wheatgrass along with other produce will take more time than it does with non-masticating juicers. Some wheatgrass-juicers are more time-consuming to clean as well.

Give wheatgrass a try by combining the ingredients in the following recipes.

Wheatgrass Light

Though wheatgrass is most effective when consumed by itself, some people just can't tolerate the taste of wheatgrass, so I designed this recipe to help. At our retreats we serve wheatgrass juice twice a day with a lemon wedge chaser or a dash of cinnamon.

1 green apple, washed
1 handful of wheatgrass, rinsed
2–3 sprigs mint, rinsed (optional)
½ lemon, washed, or peeled if not organic

Cut produce to fit your juicer's feed tube. Start with apple and juice all ingredients and stir. Pour into a glass and drink as soon as possible. Serves 1.

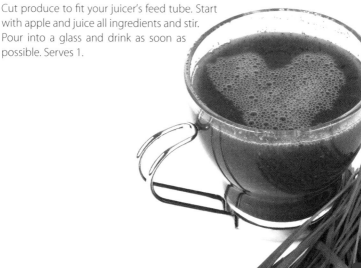

Wheatgrass With Coconut Water

1–2 ounces wheatgrass juice
8 oz. coconut water

Juice wheatgrass and pour into a glass. Add coconut water and
stir. Serves 1.

Smoothies

In addition to juicing, you can make healthy smoothies to help
manage blood sugar and improve your health. A juicer won't
make smoothies, so you will need a blender. Smoothies are a
great addition to a healthy diet because they have a creamy tex-
ture to which you can add some protein. Green smoothies (made
from nutrient-rich, dark-green vegetables) are the best for those
who are watching both their weight and the glycemic load in their
daily diets. Smoothies are ideal when you want to include ingredients such as coconut milk, protein powder, nuts, or tofu.

See chapter 7, "Helpful Recipes for Diabetes—Juices and
Smoothies," for a list of delicious juice and smoothie recipes that
will help you lose weight and stay healthy.

Chapter 6

LIVING FOODS MAKE ALL THE DIFFERENCE

I N MY BOOK *The Juice Lady's Living Foods Revolution* I explain in detail how to choose and combine "living foods" to improve and maintain health and vitality. In this chapter I want to apply what I have learned toward improvement, if not reversal, of diabetes and prediabetic conditions. Some experts claim that type 2 diabetes can be completely reversed by carefully following a low-glycemic regimen that includes juicing.[1] I am convinced that type 1 diabetics can benefit from a knowledgeable application of the same principles. I have met type 1 diabetics who have greatly improved their condition with this type of diet.

Refined and processed foods are the biggest food culprits. The body of someone who eats a lot of refined foods (which means eating a lot of sugar and refined flour products) will develop an imbalance in the hormone insulin. Over time poor eating can lead to insulin resistance and eventually diabetes. This takes years to develop, but it doesn't have to happen at all. If you start making wise food choices now, your body (and your family) will thank you forever.

Besides learning how to shop for and prepare the foods you need, you must resist the temptation to purchase ready-made juices and (especially) soda. Instead, make your own fresh juices at home! Never resort to diet sodas to help you lose weight and fight diabetes—they are more dangerous to your health than you think. The San Antonio Heart Study—a twenty-five-year community-based study carried out at the University of Texas Health Science Center in San Antonio—found that the more diet sodas a person drinks, the *greater* his chance of becoming overweight or obese, and added weight is a strong risk factor for the development of type 2 diabetes. Sharon Fowler, a faculty associate for the study, put it this way: "On average, for each diet soft drink participants drank per day, they were 65 percent more likely to become overweight during the next seven to eight years, and 41 percent more likely to become obese."[2]

What Are Living Foods?

Living foods are foods that are alive—raw (not cooked) and filled with life. They're also called raw foods or live foods. You can plant them, pick them, sprout them, or simply eat them. In each case—you get life! That's because life comes from life. These foods are your "true north," your path home to health in a jungle of dietary havoc, contaminated food, and abounding confusion about what and how to eat.

What constitutes human nourishment that blesses us with abundant health? Is it the antibiotic-laden, growth-hormone-laced flesh of stressed-out, factory-farm animals? How about pasteurized milk products with their denatured protein and damaged fats? Is it cooked or processed vegetables saturated with pesticides and preservatives? Maybe it's designer foods with "good health promises." Perhaps it's the long line of prescription pills coming out of the thunderous jaws of manufacturing plants.

My dear friends, we've been duped—completely led astray—by marketing campaigns. Good health is the result of consuming whole, unprocessed, clean food with a large percentage of that being raw and alive. These foods are chock-full of nutrients, water, and fiber that flush away toxins, waste, and "sludge" from our cells and intercellular fluids. They help us prevent disease and heal the diseases from which we suffer.

Living foods are basic foods in their uncooked form. Cooking always depletes nutrients, so it stands to reason that uncooked foods will provide more benefits. You don't have to become an all-raw foodist to benefit from them. I'm not. I am encouraging you to get more raw food in your diet and to make it a bit more than half of the food you eat every day. Juicing and green smoothies represent one way to help you reach that goal easily.

Two other terms for living or raw foods are "real foods" or "whole foods." They are the opposite of food substances that are man-made—whipped up in factories and spun out in forms that are anything but real or whole. Such foods have become the basis of the American diet, but they should not be called food and should not be part of anyone's diet. They are processed, depleted of natural nutrients, and filled with chemicals to promote longer shelf life, ease of transportation, and longer storage. After being grown in vast fields and saturated with pesticides and artificial fertilizers, plant nutrient values are further diminished in the course of processing and storage, so the processed foods must be fortified with synthetic vitamins and minerals. Flavorings are added to improve the taste because they have very little flavor left. These foods are often addictive and carcinogenic, while being void of nutrients necessary for cellular function. And they deliver empty calories that get stored as fat because the body can't use them to meet its needs. These products have made Americans the most overfed and yet undernourished nation in the world.

Real foods are the foods that are the least processed. They are closest to their natural form and, therefore, retain the most nutrient value and deliver the highest health benefits. They are most nutritious when picked after they've ripened, and they are then the richest in flavor. They retain natural diversity of taste. They have full nutrient and antioxidant content. And if they are organically grown, seasonal, and local foods, they are the healthiest choices possible.

Choosing Wisely

Ideally we could grow a large proportion of our own food and thus control every stage of the process, from soil preparation to harvest. Realistically, of course, not only is that impossible for most people in terms of available time and financial freedom, it is also beyond the limits of geography and climate. We must find reliable sources of a wide variety of foods in order to cover our nutritional needs.

I want to guide you in how to make the best food choices possible by providing you with shopping tips to help you bypass the endless options of unhealthy foodstuff that line the shelves and freezers of our supermarkets. Our mission is to choose living foods that are also clean, fresh, whole foods—foods that give our bodies life. Though I don't believe that we have to eat all raw (uncooked) foods to be healthy, I do believe we should choose whole foods that provide the nourishment we need.

Shop "smart." The majority of the food in typical grocery stores does not give the body life, therefore smart shopping is the key to healthy eating.

Plan ahead. This is the best way to avoid making poor food choices when there's nothing around to eat and you feel half starved. If you make meal plans and shop ahead of time, you'll have food on hand and an idea for when and how you'll make the food. This will give you a much better chance of succeeding with your living foods lifestyle. If something unexpected comes your way, have a backup plan to eat nutritious food you can thaw out, dehydrated foods that are already made, or a meal or snack you can quickly put together, many times in the form of a smoothie or juice.

Choose living foods. Raw juices and living foods are packed with a cornucopia of nutrients, including biophotons—those light rays of energy the plants get from the sun. When we cook food, those rays of energy are destroyed or shrink way down. The more light a food is able to store, the more beneficial the food. Naturally grown fruits and vegetables that are ripened in the sun are strong sources of light energy. Numerous minute particles of light—biophotons, the smallest units of light—make their way into our cells when we eat these foods. They provide our bodies with important information and control complex processes such as ordering and regulating our cells.[3]

When you drink a tall glass of fresh veggie juice and your day is focused on more live foods than on cooked or processed fare, your whole internal environment changes. As you consume more living foods, you require fewer calories because biophotons help rev up the mitochondria of your cells—the little energy furnaces that pump out adenosine triphosphate (ATP), the energy that is used by cells. They also feed your DNA, which stores about 90 percent of the biophotons found in your cells. Because biophotons carry the biological information of the plant into your body, it's kind of like getting a software download or having a computer technician take over your computer remotely to fix things you can't begin to correct on your own. Just as the computer tech fixes errors on your computer, the biophotons help to fix errors that have taken place within the body.[4]

EAT A VARIETY OF FOODS

Raw foods are helpful for their superior nutrients, but if you are not a vegan, you can choose a combination of raw foods, some cooked foods, and some animal products that are organic, grass-fed, and free range. Eat lots of high-fiber vegetables and look for high-quality protein sources. You may need some animal protein unless you go mostly raw and really focus on getting enough high-quality protein from seeds, nuts, sprouts, and dark leafy greens.

Opt for the freshest food you can find that has been grown organically in order to obtain the very best fruits, vegetables, and legumes; avoid toxic pesticides; and get increased nutrition.

Buy from local growers whenever possible. Their produce is fresher than anything trucked in from other locations. Many local growers will deliver a box of produce to your door each week; check out websites for organic growers in your area. And if you select the produce in season, that's about the freshest food you'll be able to find. Vegetables and fruit selected off the shelf at a grocery store usually emit fewer biophotons because of loss during transportation and storage. Chemical, gas, or heat treatment, which is used to ripen or preserve fruits and vegetables, further reduces the amount of biophotons and nutrients available. Irradiation, which is radiation treatment with gamma rays in order to increase the shelf life of food, leads to total destruction of biophotons and many nutrients. We might be buying attractive fruits and veggies at the market, but their biophoton, enzyme, and vitamin content may be close to zero. For example, avocados may be heat treated in order to speed up ripening, but if the heat is above 118 degrees, it kills enzymes, vitamins, and biophotons—the life force of the cells. Most almonds are required to be pasteurized, but even raw almonds may actually have undergone pasteurization, thereby eliminating their biophoton content and reducing their nutrients.

LIGHT AFFECTS NUTRIENTS

When you shop at a store, do you select your produce from the front of a display or do you reach to the back, hoping that's the freshest and least picked over? If you think the hidden produce is the best, a new study may convince you to select your fruits and veggies differently. The U.S. Department of Agriculture (USDA) scientists recommend that consumers select their produce 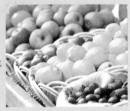 from those receiving the greatest light—usually found to the front or top of the display. For example, researchers found that spinach that was exposed to continuous light during storage was more nutritionally dense than the spinach that was continually in the dark. The scientists said that light affects the leaves' photosynthetic system, which resulted in an increase in vitamins C, E, K, and folic acid.[5]

Shop at farmers' markets. The freshest produce can be found at farmers' markets, local farms, and your own backyard, along with foraging wild greens. It may be that the healthiest food we can find will be unsprayed dandelions in our own backyard.

The quality of protein in vegetables is related to the amount of nitrogen in the soil. Conventional chemical fertilizers add extra nitrogen, which increases the amount of protein but creates a reduction in its quality. Organically managed soils release nitrogen in smaller amounts over a longer time than conventional fertilizers. As a result, the quality of protein from organic crops is better in terms of human nutrition. Indeed, studies show that across the board, organically grown produce is higher in nutrients.[6]

Choose heirloom and wild plants as often as possible. The more of these plants that we eat, the more high-quality nutrition we get. Wild foods such as dandelion greens, nettles, burdock, wood sorrel, wild salad greens, and shepherd's purse offer us nutrients found nowhere else. Consider also that if people have adapted to eating wild plants for several hundred thousand years, then problems may arise when we try to eat hybridized and genetically engineered fruits and veggies. Our physiology is just not programmed to handle this.

When commercial plants are hybridized, they lose more and more of their inherent biological information contained in the DNA. This is what also makes them more susceptible to the onslaught of diseases, insects, and parasites. Then farmers are told they need to spray their crops with highly toxic chemicals to kill the pests. It's a destructive cycle that affects our health in the end. The more nutrient-rich foods you eat, the more satisfied you'll be and the more cravings will diminish. That will have a positive impact on your health and weight management. (Also, this will have positive benefits for farmworkers, the animals, and our earth.)

Purchase lots of brightly colored vegetables. They are packed with satisfying nutrients. Eat plenty of soups, salads, sprouts, vegetable sticks, and steamed vegetables, along with drinking veggie juices and green smoothies and eating raw food dishes. Avoid baked vegetables as much as possible since baking caramelizes the sugars, creating the highest sugar content possible. Limit high-starch vegetables such as potatoes, yams, and winter squash to no more than three times per week until you get your blood sugar controlled. If you're dining out or it's a special occasion, and you just can't resist a potato, the best choice is red potatoes (lower carbohydrates). If you do succumb to a baked potato, which is very high in carbs, eat it with a little fat such as butter. This will help to slow down the rate at which sugar enters your blood stream.

Bring home some low-sugar fruit. Seven of the best fruits you can choose are lemons, limes, avocados, tomatoes, green apples, berries, and cranberries. Avocados are an excellent source of essential fatty acids and glutathione (a powerful antioxidant), along with some protein. They contain more potassium than bananas. Tomatoes are a rich source of vitamin C, beta-carotene, potassium, molybdenum, and one of the best sources of lycopene. The antioxidant function of lycopene includes its ability to help protect cells and other structures in the body from oxygen damage. It has been linked in human research to the protection of DNA inside of white blood cells. To get the most lycopene, choose organic tomatoes.

To avoid getting too much sugar, choose the lowest glycemic fruit. Besides lemons, limes, and cranberries, look for other berries, dark cherries, grapefruit, and apples (especially green). Purchase organic fruits only because so many of them are heavily sprayed. Beware of eating too much fruit except for lemons, limes, avocados, tomatoes, and cranberries. You can buy cranberries in the fall and freeze some (right in their bags) for when they're out of season. If you buy store-bought cranberry juice, look for unsweetened cranberry concentrate or pure unsweetened cranberry juice. (Of the bottled juices, cranberry contains the least amount of fungus.) Add lemon, lime, or cranberry juice to flavor water and other juices.

Buy Organic

It is important that you choose organic produce whenever possible. The popularity of organic foods continues to grow, and it is becoming more available as a result. I'm often asked if organic produce is more nutritious than conventionally grown produce. Studies have shown that it is. According to results from the largest study of organic food to date, organic produce completely outshines conventional produce in nutritional content. A four-year, European-Union-funded study found that organic fruits and vegetables contain up to 40 percent more antioxidants, that they have higher levels of beneficial minerals such as iron and zinc, and that milk from organic herds contains up to 90 percent more antioxidants. The researchers obtained their results after growing fruits and vegetables and raising cattle on adjacent organic and nonorganic sites. Eating organic foods can even help to increase the nutrient intake of people who don't eat the recommended number of servings of fruits and vegetables a day.[7]

When choosing organically grown foods, look for labels that are marked "certified organic." This means the produce has been cultivated according to strict uniform standards that are verified by independent state or private organizations. Certification includes the following: inspection of farms and processing facilities, detailed record-keeping, and pesticide-testing of soil and water to ensure that growers and handlers are meeting government standards. You may occasionally see a label that says transitional organic. This means that the produce was grown on a farm that recently converted, or is in the process of converting, from chemical sprays and fertilizer to organic farming.

Support your local farms and farmers who sell their produce at farmers' markets, local markets, and home deliveries. Many of the smaller farms can't promote their wares as "organic" because they can't afford certification, but if you talk with them, you'll learn that they don't use pesticides or chemical fertilizers.

You may not be able to afford to purchase everything organic. When that's the case, choose wisely. According to the Environmental Working Group commercially farmed fruits and vegetables vary in their levels of pesticide residue. Some vegetables—broccoli, asparagus, and onions, for example—as well as foods with thicker peels (which you remove) have relatively low levels of pesticides compared to other fruits and vegetables.[8]

TWO FOODS THAT ARE A MUST-BUY ORGANIC

Potatoes are a staple of the American diet, up to 30 percent of our overall vegetable consumption. Switching to organic potatoes can potentially have a big impact because commercially farmed potatoes are some of the most pesticide-contaminated vegetables. The potato has one of the highest pesticide contents of the forty-three fruits and vegetables tested by the Environmental Working Group.

Apples are the second most commonly eaten fresh fruit, after bananas, and they are the second most popular fruit juice, after oranges. But apples are also one of the most pesticide-contaminated fruits. The good news is that organic apples are easy to find and readily available in most grocery stores and big-box stores.[9]

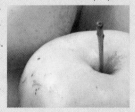

When organic vegetables or fruits that you want are not available, ask your grocer to get them. You can also look for small-operation farmers in your area and check out farmers' markets in season. Many owners of small farms can't afford to use as many chemicals in farming as large commercial farms use, so even if their produce isn't certified organic, it is healthier than what you will find in a store.

Organic produce from Mexico

What about Mexican organics? In the winter, when fresh produce is not available in most parts of the United States, we see grocers' shelves stocked with produce displaying Mexican "certified organic" stickers. How many times have you wondered if this is reliable organic produce? It appears that this produce is as reliable as US-grown organics. For a food to be sold in the United States, Mexico, or anywhere else, and to be labeled organic, it must meet all the requirements of the USDA National Organics Program. This means it must be produced without the use of synthetic pesticides, artificial fertilizers, sewage sludge, genetically modified organisms, or irradiation. And it must be certified by a USDA-accredited agency to be labeled organic.

Certification includes inspection of farms and processing facilities, detailed record-keeping of whatever is applied to the land, and, if there's cause for concern, water-testing. Currently there are fifteen organic certification agencies in Mexico. Plus, the USDA has begun more border inspections to ensure food safety.

Supporting Mexican organic farmers is a part of compassionate eating. By purchasing fresh organic produce from Mexico that is not available locally in off seasons, we are supporting small farmers who earn a wage, such as those who sell products recognized as "fair trade," and empowering them to stay on their land and remain in their communities rather than leaving home to seek employment.

In the next chapter the juice and smoothie recipes were created almost exclusively with living foods, and most of them contain more vegetables than fruit. The vegetables and fruits included are primarily low glycemic. However, you may change any of the recipes to fit your needs. If there is something you are allergic to in a recipe, omit it or substitute another food. If your blood sugar is not yet under control, you may need to omit almost all fruit, with the exception of lemons, limes, and cranberries. (Lemon is a nice addition to almost any recipe.) All other berries and green apples are next in line as the fruits lowest in sugar.

Chapter 7

HELPFUL RECIPES FOR DIABETES—JUICES AND SMOOTHIES

I N THE PAGES that follow you'll discover a wide variety of juices and smoothies. Some are basic juice recipes for those who are just getting started and want something simple. Most fruity juices contain fruits that have lower-than-average glycemic values. Green juices (my favorites) are in a separate category and offer the most nutrition of all. These recipes have been modified for diabetic use.

Some of the recipes may include fruits or vegetables with a higher glycemic level in order to sweeten the otherwise very "green"-tasting juice. If you are having difficulty keeping your blood sugar stable, try those recipes without the questionable ingredient; you may not miss it as much as you think you would.

To be safe, keep your juices as low in sugar as possible. Often the green leafy vegetables and high-water-content veggies such as cucumbers will be enough to offset the sugar content of a small amount of fruit or sweet vegetable. Green beans, for example, are good for the pancreas and help stabilize blood sugar levels. However, if a recipe contains all or mostly fruit— even low-glycemic fruit—it may be necessary for you to avoid it until your blood sugar is stabilized and your body is processing such foods in a normal manner.

Juices

Arugula Lemon Juice

1 cucumber, peeled if not organic
1 lemon, peeled if not organic
1 green apple
1 small handful of arugula

Cut all ingredients to fit your juicer's feed tube and push through the juicer. Stir and serve as soon as possible. Serves 1.

Berry Bright Eyes

Berries are rich in antioxidants that help fight degenerative eye disorders. They also help improve vision. You can also help prevent eye disorders by avoiding sugar; it promotes swelling of the lenses and increases the risk of free-radical damage to the eyes.

1 Celestial Seasonings Wild Berry Zinger herbal tea bag
½ cup fresh or frozen (thawed) blackberries
½ cup fresh or frozen (thawed) blueberries
1 handful of spinach

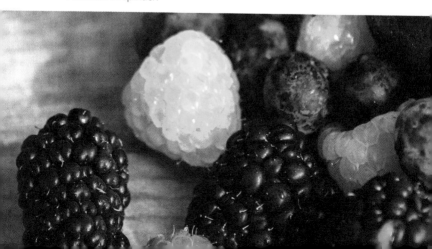

1 dark green lettuce leaf
¼ tsp. pure raspberry extract

Steep one bag of Wild Berry Zinger herbal tea in a cup of hot water for about twenty minutes, or until the tea is strong and flavorful. Set aside to cool. With the juicer off, pour in the berries. Turn the machine on and juice. Wrap the spinach in the lettuce leaf and push through the juicer slowly. Combine with herbal tea and raspberry extract. Stir and serve as soon as soon possible. Serves 1–2.

Black Currant-Lemon-Apple

2 green apples
½ lemon, peeled if not organic
1 cup fresh black currants

Cut produce to fit your juicer's feed tube. Juice one apple and lemon. Turn off machine, add currants and then the plunger. Turn machine back on and push the currants through. Follow with the second apple and stir the juice. Pour into a glass and served chilled. Serves 1.

Blueberry-Apple Juice

1 cup blueberries, fresh or frozen (thawed)
2 green apples

Cut apples to fit your juicer's feed tube. With the machine off, pour in the berries and top with the plunger, which will keep the berries from flying out. Then turn the machine on and push the berries through followed by the apples. Stir the juice and pour into a glass; drink as soon as possible. Serves 1.

Butternut Squash and Apple Juice

4–5 strips of raw butternut squash, cut in strips ½ inch by 4 inches
1 apple
1–2 kale leaves
2 ribs of celery with leaves
1-inch-chunk of ginger

Cut produce to fit your juicer's feed tube. Juice ingredients and stir. Pour into a glass and drink as soon as possible. Serves 1.

Caliente Fiesta

1 cucumber, peeled if not organic
2-inch by 4- or 5-inch chunk of jicama, scrubbed or peeled if not organic
¼ small jalapeño, seeds removed unless you like it hot

Cut produce to fit your juicer's feed tube. Juice ingredients and stir. Pour into a glass and drink as soon as possible. Serves 1.

Chili Lime

2- or 3-inch by 4- or 5-inch chunk of jicama, scrubbed or peeled if not organic
1 lime, peeled if not organic
¼ small jalapeño, seeds removed unless you like it hot

Cut produce to fit your juicer's feed tube. Juice ingredients and stir. Pour into a glass and drink as soon as possible. Serves 1.

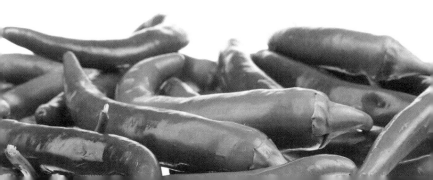

Cilantro-Mint-Jalapeño

1 cucumber, peeled if not organic
1 bunch of spearmint
1 bunch of cilantro
1 lime, peeled
¼ jalapeño pepper, seeds removed unless you like it hot

Cut all ingredients to fit your juicer's feed tube and push through the juicer, stir and serve as soon as possible. Serves 1.

Cran-Apple Cocktail

2 organic green apples
¼–½ cup fresh or frozen (thawed) cranberries
½ cucumber, peeled if not organic
½ lemon, peeled if not organic
1-inch-chunk of ginger
¼ cup purified water (optional)

Cut produce to fit your juicer's feed tube. Juice one apple first. Turn off the machine, add the cranberries, and put the plunger in; then turn the machine on and juice. Follow with the lemon, ginger, and second apple. Add water as needed. Stir and pour into a glass; drink as soon as possible. Serves 1–2.

Cranberry-Pear Fat Blaster

Studies show that cranberries boost metabolism and their acids help dissolve fat. In addition, cranberries are a diuretic, so they help you get rid of stored up water. They also have soluble fiber, which is not entirely lost with juicing. (Note: Use this recipe only when you have your blood sugar under control because of the pear. However, you can make this recipe right away omitting the pear.)

2 pears, Bartlett or Asian
½ cucumber, peeled if not organic
¼ lemon, peeled if not organic

2 Tbsp. cranberries, fresh or thawed if frozen
½- to 1-inch-chunk of gingerroot

Cut produce to fit your juicer's feed tube. Juice all ingredients and stir. Pour into a glass and drink as soon as possible. Serves 1–2.

Cucumber Dill

1 cucumber, peeled if not organic
1 lime, peeled if not organic
2 sprigs fresh dill

Cut produce to fit your juicer's feed tube. Juice ingredients and stir. Pour into a glass and drink as soon as possible. Serves 1.

Cucumber Lime Cooler

1 cucumber
1 lime, peeled if not organic

Cut produce to fit your juicer's feed tube. Juice ingredients and stir. Pour over ice and drink as soon as possible. Serves 1.

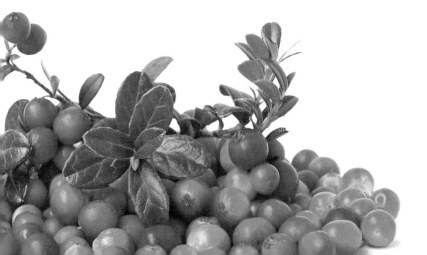

Cucumber-Tomato-Cilantro Cooler

1 cucumber, peeled if not organic
2 tomatoes
1 handful of cilantro
1 lime, peeled if not organic

Cut all ingredients to fit your juicers feed tube and push through the juicer. Pour over ice, stir, and serve chilled. Serves 2.

Elderberry-Strawberry-Apple

1 green apple
1 cup elderberries
1 cup strawberries with caps

Cut produce to fit your juicer's feed tube. Juice the apple. Turn off the machine and add the elderberries and top with the plunger. Push berries through and add the strawberries. Stir the juice and pour into a glass; serve chilled. Serves 1.

Fennel-Apple

Fennel juice has been used as a traditional tonic to help the body release endorphins, the "feel good" peptides from the brain into the bloodstream. Endorphins help to diminish anxiety and fear and generate a happy mood.

¼ fennel bulb with fronds
1–2 green apples

Cut produce to fit your juicer's feed tube. Juice ingredients and stir. Pour into a glass and drink as soon as possible. Serves 1.

Fennel-Watercress-Cucumber

1 handful of watercress
1 dark green lettuce leaf
1 cucumber, peeled if not organic

½ fennel bulb and fronds
1 lemon, peeled if not organic

Cut produce to fit your juicer's feed tube. Wrap watercress in lettuce leaf and push through juicer slowly. Juice all remaining ingredients. Pour into a glass, stir, and drink as soon as possible. Serves 1.

Four-Veggie Supreme

2 tomatoes
1 fennel bulb with fronds
2 ribs of celery with leaves
1 handful of flat-leaf parsley
½ tsp. Celtic sea salt

Cut produce to fit your juicer's feed tube. Juice ingredients and stir. Pour into a glass, stir in the salt, and drink as soon as possible. Serves 1.

Fresh Fennel

2 fennel bulbs with fronds
2 ribs of celery with leaves
1 pear or green apple

Cut produce to fit your juicer's feed tube. Juice all ingredients. Pour into a glass and drink as soon as possible. Serves 1.

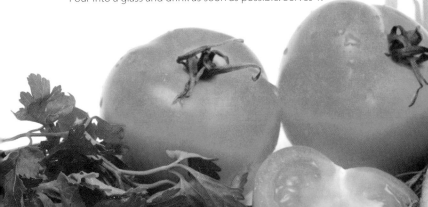

Fresh Pink Morning

1 large pink grapefruit, peeled
½ green apple
1-inch-chunk of fresh ginger, peeled

Cut produce to fit your juicer's feed tube. Juice all ingredients and stir. Pour into a glass and drink as soon as possible. Serves 1.

Green Apple-Celery

2 green apples
4 ribs of celery with leaves

Cut produce to fit your juicer's feed tube. Juice ingredients and stir. Pour into a glass and drink as soon as possible. Serves 1.

Green Apple-Cucumber Cooler

1 cucumber
1 green apple
½ lemon, peeled if not organic

Cut produce to fit your juicer's feed tube. Juice ingredients and stir. Pour over ice and drink as soon as possible. Serves 1.

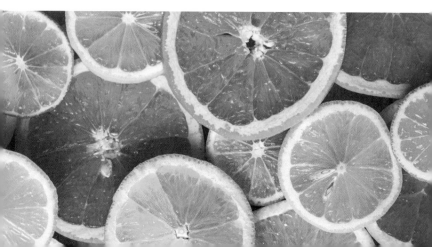

Grapefruit, Fennel, and Spring Greens

½ fennel bulb with fronds
1 handful of spring greens
1 red grapefruit, peeled

Cut produce to fit your juicer's feed tube. Juice ingredients and stir. Pour into a glass and drink as soon as possible. Serves 1.

Grapefruit-Strawberry Sparkler

1 grapefruit, peeled
1 lime, peeled
10 strawberries with caps
1 cup chilled sparkling water

Cut produce to fit your juicer's feed tube. Juice all ingredients and stir in sparkling water. Pour into a glass and served chilled. Serves 2.

Happy Mary

1 large cucumber, peeled if not organic
1 tomato
3 ribs of celery with leaves
1 lemon, peeled if not organic
⅛ tsp. hot sauce
Pinch Celtic sea salt
Pinch black pepper

Cut produce to fit your juicer's feed tube. Juice cucumbers, tomato, celery, and lemon. Stir in hot sauce, salt, and pepper. Serve chilled over ice. Serves 2.

Jicama Delight

2-inch by 4- or 5-inch chunk of jicama, scrubbed well or peeled
½ green apple
½ cucumber, peeled if not organic
¼ daikon radish, trimmed and scrubbed
1-inch-chunk of ginger, scrubbed, peeled if old
½ lemon or lime, peeled if not organic

Cut produce to fit your juicer's feed tube. Juice all ingredients and stir. Pour into a glass and drink as soon as possible. Serves 1.

La Florentine

2 tomatoes
1 large handful of spinach
4 or 5 sprigs of basil
1 lemon, peeled if not organic
½ cucumber, peeled if not organic

Juice one tomato. Wrap the basil in several spinach leaves. Turn off the machine and add the spinach and basil. Turn the machine back on and gently tap to juice them. Juice the remaining ingredients. Stir juice, pour in a glass and drink as soon as possible. Serves 1.

Lemon-Fennel on Ice

1 fennel bulb with fronds
1 cucumber, peeled if not organic
1 lemon, peeled if not organic

Cut produce to fit your juicer's feed tube. Juice all ingredients and serve chilled, over ice. Serves 2.

Lemon-Lime-Blueberry

1 cucumber, peeled if not organic
1 green apple
1 cup fresh or frozen (thawed) blueberries
½ lemon, peeled if not organic
½ lime, peeled if not organic

Cut produce to fit your juicer's feed tube. Juice the cucumber and apple. Turn off the machine and add the blueberries and top with the plunger. Push berries through and juice the lemon and lime. Stir the juice and pour into a glass; serve chilled. Serves 1.

Lemon-Lime Slushy

Juice of two limes
Juice of one lemon
4–6 drops of stevia
1½ cups sparkling water
Ice

Mix the juice with the stevia and sparkling water. Pour into two tall glasses over ice and serve chilled. Serves 2.

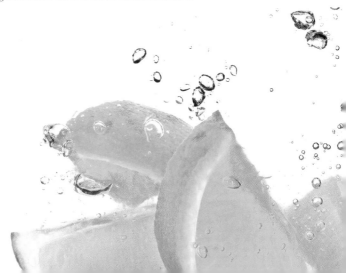

Lime Cordial

2 green apples
1 lime, peeled if not organic
1–2 drops of stevia
1 cup sparkling water

Juice the apples and lime. Pour into a glass and add the stevia and sparkling water. Add ice. Stir and drink as soon as possible. Serves 1.

Magnesium-Rich Cocktail

A study out of the University of North Carolina at Chapel Hill points to a connection between magnesium in the diet and lowered risk of diabetes.[1]

4–5 beet tops
2 Swiss chard leaves
2 collard leaves
1 cucumber, peeled if not organic
½ cup blueberries, thawed if frozen
½ lemon, peeled if not organic

Cut produce to fit your juicer's feed tube. Turn off the machine when adding the blueberries. Put the plunger in place, then turn the machine on and juice, followed by the lemon. Stir. Pour into a glass and drink as soon as possible. Serves 2.

Plain Janie

1 green apple
1 cup strawberries with caps

Cut produce to fit your juicer's feed tube. Juice all ingredients and stir. Pour into a glass and served chilled. Serves 1.

Quince and Spice

1 large quince
1 green apple
1 lemon, peeled if not organic
Dash of cinnamon
Dash of nutmeg

Cut produce to fit your juicer's feed tube. Juice ingredients and stir in cinnamon and nutmeg. Pour into a glass and drink as soon as possible. Serves 1.

Raspberry Limeade

2 green apples
1 lime, peeled 1 cup
    raspberries

Cut produce to fit your juicer's feed tube. Juice one apple and the lime. Turn off the machine and add the raspberries and top with the plunger. Push berries through and add the remaining apple. Stir the juice and pour into a glass; serve chilled. Serves 1.

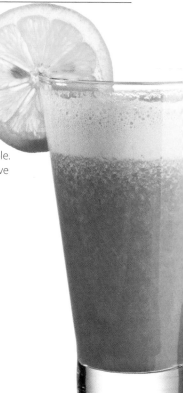

Razz and Spazz

1 green apple
1 lime, peeled
1 cup fresh or frozen (thawed) raspberries
½ cucumber, peeled if not organic
¼ cup fresh mint leaves

Cut produce to fit your juicer's feed tube. Juice apple and lime. Turn off the machine and add the raspberries and top with the plunger. Push berries through and add the remaining apple, cucumber, and mint. Stir the juice and pour into a glass; serve chilled. Serves 1.

Red Sunset

1 blood orange, peeled
4 purple kale leaves
¼ red cabbage
1 lemon, peeled if not organic
½ beet with leaves
¼ bunch mint
1-inch-chunk of ginger

Cut produce to fit your juicer's feed tube. Juice ingredients and stir. Pour into a glass and drink as soon as possible. Serves 2.

Refreshing Mint Cocktail

2 fennel stalks with fronds
1 cucumber, peeled if not organic
1 green apple such as Granny Smith or Pippin
1 handful of mint
1-inch-chunk of gingerroot

Cut produce to fit your juicer's feed tube. Juice all ingredients and stir. Pour into a glass and drink as soon as possible. Serves 1–2.

Refreshing Mint Cooler

1 fennel bulb and fronds
1 cucumber, peeled if not organic
1 green apple
1 handful of mint

Cut produce to fit your juicer's feed tube. Juice ingredients and stir. Pour into a glass over ice and drink as soon as possible. Serves 1–2.

Rockin' Tomato

1 cup loosely packed flat-leaf parsley
1 dark green lettuce leaf
2 tomatoes
1 fennel bulb with fronds
2 celery ribs with leaves
1 green onion
Pinch of Celtic sea salt

Cut produce to fit your juicer's feed tube. Wrap parsley in lettuce leaf. Juice remaining ingredients and stir. Pour into a glass and drink as soon as possible. Serves 2.

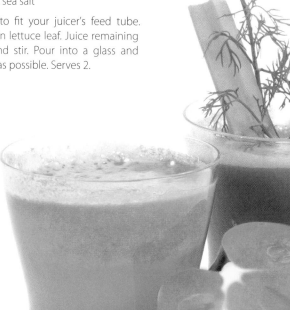

Santa Fe Salsa Cocktail

1 medium tomato
1 cucumber, peeled if not organic
1 small handful of cilantro
1 lime, peeled
Dash of hot sauce or ¼ jalapeño pepper (optional)

Cut produce to fit your juicer's feed tube. Juice ingredients and stir. Pour into a glass and drink as soon as possible. Serves 1.

Siesta Refresher

4 sprigs parsley
2 dark green lettuce leaves
2 medium tomatoes
2 radishes, with leaves
1 lime, peeled if not organic

Cut produce to fit your juicer's feed tube. Wrap parsley in lettuce and push through juicer slowly. Juice remaining ingredients and stir. Pour into a glass and drink as soon as possible. Serves 1.

South of the Border Cocktail

1 medium tomato
1 cucumber, peeled if not organic
1 handful cilantro
1 lime, peeled if not organic
Dash of hot sauce (optional)

Cut produce to fit your juicer's feed tube. Juice all ingredients and stir. Pour into a glass and drink as soon as possible. Serves 1.

Southwest Spicy Tomato

1 small handful of cilantro
1 small handful of parsley
2 dark green lettuce leaves
2 medium tomatoes
1 lime, peeled if not organic
½ jalapeño, seeds removed unless you like it hot

Cut produce to fit your juicer's feed tube. Wrap cilantro and parsley in lettuce leaves and push through the juicer slowly. Juice remaining ingredients and stir. Pour into two glasses and drink as soon as possible. Serves 2.

Squash Blossom Surprise

3–4 squash blossoms
1 large heirloom tomato
4 sprigs fresh basil
2 ribs of celery with leaves

Cut produce to fit your juicer's feed tube. Juice ingredients and stir. Pour into a glass and drink as soon as possible. Serves 1.

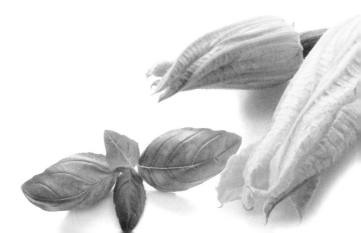

Strawberry-Mint Cordial

    1 pint strawberries with caps
    1 handful of mint
    1–2 drops of stevia
    1 cup sparkling water

Juice the strawberries and mint. Pour in a glass and add the stevia and sparkling water, stir. Add ice. Drink as soon as possible. Serves 1.

Tomatillo Salsa Cocktail

    5–6 fresh tomatillos
    1 handful of cilantro
    1 lime, peeled if not organic
    1 garlic clove
    ¼ small jalapeño pepper, seeds removed unless you like it really
        hot

Cut produce to fit your juicer's feed. Juice all ingredients and stir. Pour into a glass and drink as soon as possible. Serves 1.

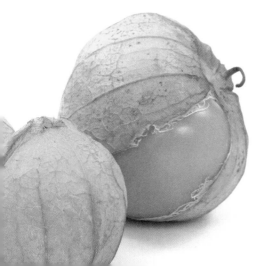

Tomato-Cucumber-Dill

2 tomatoes
1 cucumber, peeled if not organic
1 stalk fresh dill weed

Cut produce to fit your juicer's feed. Juice all ingredients and stir. Pour into a glass and drink as soon as possible. Serves 1.

Veggie Delight

1 cucumber, peeled
2–3 ribs of celery with leaves
½ organic lemon, with peel
1-inch-chunk of gingerroot

Cut produce to fit your juicer's feed tube. Juice ingredients and stir. Pour into a glass and drink as soon as possible. Serves 1–2.

Virgin Mary

2 tomatoes
2 ribs of celery with leaves
1 lemon, peeled if not organic
Dash of hot sauce
Dash of black pepper
Dash of Celtic sea salt

Cut produce to fit your juicer's feed tube. Juice ingredients and stir in hot sauce, pepper, and salt. Pour into a glass of ice and drink as soon as possible. Serves 1.

Waldorf Twist

1 green apple
3 ribs of organic celery with leaves
1 lemon, peeled if not organic

Cut produce to fit your juicer's feed tube. Juice all ingredients and stir. Pour into a glass and drink as soon as possible. Serves 1.

Green Juices

Broccoli Surprise

2–3 broccoli florets or 1 broccoli stem
1 carrot, scrubbed well, top removed, end trimmed
2 ribs of celery with leaves
1 cucumber, peeled if not organic
1 lemon, peeled if not organic

Cut produce to fit your juicer's feed tube. Juice all ingredients, stir, and drink as soon as possible. Serves 1.

Brussels Delight

3 brussels sprouts
1 large vine-ripened tomato
2 romaine lettuce leaves
8 organic string beans
½ small or medium lemon, peeled

Cut produce to fit your juicer's feed tube. Juice ingredients and stir. Pour into a glass and drink as soon as possible. Serves 1.

Dandelion-Coconut Water

Dandelion greens are quite bitter; you can sweeten them with a lower-sugar fruit such as green apple or pear.

1 bunch dandelion greens
1 lime, peeled if not organic
1 cup coconut water, unsweetened

Juice the dandelion greens and lime, stir in coconut water, and serve immediately. Serves 1.

Dino Delight

4–5 leaves dino kale
1 cucumber, peeled if not organic
1 green apple

Cut all ingredients to fit your juicers feed tube and push through the juicer, stir, and serve as soon as possible. Serves 1.

Energize-Your-Day Cocktail

1 green apple
2 dark green leaves (chard, collard, or kale)
1 rib of celery with leaves
1 lemon, peeled if not organic
½ cucumber, peeled if not organic
½- to 1-inch-chunk of fresh gingerroot, peeled

Cut the apple into sections that fit your juicer's feed tube. Roll the green leaves and push through the feed tube with the apple, celery, lemon, cucumber, and ginger. Stir the juice and pour into a glass. Drink as soon as possible. Serves 1.

Field of Greens

3 romaine lettuce leaves
2 ribs of celery with leaves
2 kale leaves
1 green apple or 1 pear
1 lemon, peeled if not organic

Cut all ingredients to fit your juicers feed tube and push through the juicer, stir, and serve as soon as possible. Serves 1.

Green Bean Pro

2 carrots, scrubbed well, tops removed, ends trimmed
1 handful of fresh green beans
2 ribs of celery with leaves
1 cucumber, scrubbed well
1 lemon, peeled if not organic

Cut produce to fit your juicer's feed tube. Juice all ingredients, stir, and drink as soon as possible. Serves 1.

Green Delight

1 handful of parsley
1 handful of spinach
2 chard leaves
1 rib of celery with leaves
1 apple (green is lower in sugar)
½ lemon, peeled

Cut produce to fit your juicer's feed tube. Wrap the parsley and spinach in the chard leaves and push through the juicer with the celery. Juice the apple and lemon. Stir the juice and drink as soon as possible. Serves 1.

Green Goddess

2 ribs of celery with leaves
1 cucumber, peeled if not organic
3 leaves dino kale
1 fennel stalk with fronds
6 sprigs parsley

Cut produce to fit your juicer's feed tube. Juice ingredients and stir. Pour into a glass and drink as soon as possible. Serves 1.

Green Supreme

1 handful of parsley
1 small handful of cilantro
1 chard leaf
2 ribs of celery with leaves
1 cucumber, peeled if not organic
1 green apple
1 lemon, peeled if not organic
1-inch-chunk ginger root

Cut produce to fit your juicer's feed tube. Wrap parsley and cilantro in chard leaf. Start with celery and cucumber, push the lettuce-parsley-cilantro wrap through slowly and follow with remaining ingredients. Pour into a glass and drink as soon as possible. Serves 2.

Greens for Life

4 ribs of celery with leaves
4 kale leaves
1 green apple
1 cucumber, peeled if not organic
1-inch-chunk of gingerroot
1 lemon, peeled if not organic

Cut produce to fit your juicer's feed tube. Juice ingredients and stir. Pour into a glass and drink as soon as possible. Serves 1.

Healthy Bones Cocktail

Kale and parsley are loaded with calcium, magnesium, boron, and vitamin K—all important for bone health.

1 cucumber, peeled if not organic
1 large kale leaf
1 chard leaf
1 handful of parsley
1 rib of celery
1 lemon, peeled if not organic
1-inch-chunk of ginger, scrubbed or peeled if old

Cut produce to fit your juicer's feed tube. Juice all ingredients and stir. Pour into a glass and drink as soon as possible. Serves 1.

La Bella

½ green pepper with seeds
½ red pepper with seeds
3 ribs of celery with leaves
1 cucumber, peeled if not organic
4 romaine lettuce leaves

Cut produce to fit your juicer's feed tube. Juice all ingredients and stir. Pour into a glass and drink as soon as possible. Serves 2.

Lean Mean Green Juice

1 handful of parsley
1 handful of spinach
2 kale leaves
2 ribs of celery with leaves
1 cucumber, peeled if not organic
1-inch-chunk of ginger
½ green apple

Cut produce to fit your juicer's feed tube. Wrap parsley and spinach in kale leaves. Start with celery and cucumber; then push the kale wraps through slowly and follow with remaining ingredients. Pour into a glass and drink as soon as possible. Serves 2.

Lettuce Wrap

1 handful of spinach
1 small handful of parsley
2 green leaf lettuce leaves
3 ribs of celery with leaves
2 stems asparagus
1 large tomato

Cut produce to fit your juicer's feed tube. Wrap spinach and parsley in lettuce leaves. Start with celery, then juice lettuce wraps, followed by asparagus and tomato. Stir and pour into a glass; drink as soon as possible. Serves 1.

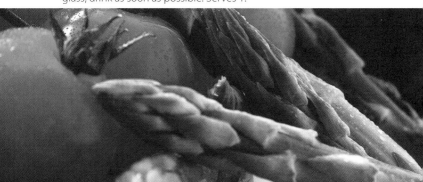

Magnesium Special

  4–5 beet tops
  2 Swiss chard leaves
  2 collard leaves
  1 cucumber, peeled if not organic
  ½ green apple
  ½ lemon, peeled if not organic

Cut produce to fit your juicer's feed tube. Juice ingredients and stir. Pour into a glass and drink as soon as possible. Serves 2.

Multi-Sprout Drink

  1 cucumber, peeled if not organic
  2 ribs of celery with leaves
  1 small handful of sprouts such as broccoli or radish
  1 large handful of sunflower sprouts
  1 small handful of buckwheat sprouts
  1 lemon, peeled if not organic

Cut produce to fit your juicer's feed tube. Juice ingredients and stir. Pour into a glass and drink as soon as possible. Serves 1.

Peppy Parsley

  1 cucumber, peeled if not organic
  1 carrot, scrubbed well, green top removed, end trimmed
  1 rib of celery with leaves
  1 handful of parsley
  1 kale leaf
  1 lemon, peeled if not organic

Cut produce to fit your juicer's feed tube. Juice the cucumber, carrot, and celery. Bunch up parsley and roll in kale leaf; add to juicer and push through. Then add lemon and juice. Stir and pour into a glass. Drink as soon as possible. Serves 1.

Rio Fiesta

1 lime, peeled if not organic
4 romaine lettuce leaves
½ small jicama, peeled if not organic
4 red radishes, with leaves

Cut produce to fit your juicer's feed tube. Start with lime and juice all ingredients and stir. Pour into a glass and drink as soon as possible. Serves 1.

Simply Green Juice

4 kale leaves
1 handful of spinach
1 handful of parsley
3 ribs of celery with leaves
1 cucumber, peeled if not organic
1 clove garlic

Cut produce to fit your juicer's feed tube. Wrap spinach and parsley in the kale leaves. Start with half the cucumber, then push the kale wraps through slowly, and follow with remaining ingredients and stir. Pour into a glass and drink as soon as possible. Serves 1.

Spicy Spinach-Grapefruit

1 cup fresh loosely packed baby spinach
1 lettuce leaf
¼ medium jicama, peeled if not organic
½ red grapefruit, peeled
1-inch-chunk of ginger

Cut produce to fit your juicer's feed tube. Wrap spinach in the lettuce leaf. Start with jicama, then push the lettuce wrap through slowly, and follow with remaining ingredients and stir. Juice ingredients and stir. Pour into a glass and drink as soon as possible. Serves 1.

Spring Greens Sprout Cocktail

3 fennel stalks with fronds
1 handful of wild chicory leaves
1 handful of mixed spring greens
½ cup broccoli sprouts
3 ribs of celery with leaves

Cut produce to fit your juicer's feed tube. Juice ingredients and stir. Pour into a glass and drink as soon as possible. Serves 1.

Springtime Tonic

Asparagus is a natural diuretic, which helps flush toxins from the body. This recipe is a great way to use up asparagus stems. You can break off the asparagus tips and steam them, saving only the tougher ends for juicing.

1 tomato
1 cucumber, peeled if not organic
8 asparagus stems
1 handful of wild greens
1 lemon, peeled if not organic

Cut produce to fit your juicer's feed tube. Juice all ingredients and stir. Pour into a glass and drink as soon as possible. Serves 1–2.

Sprout-Cucumber Recharger

1 cucumber, peeled if not organic
1 large handful of spinach
2 kale leaves
1 handful of sunflower sprouts (optional)
1 handful of buckwheat sprouts (optional)
1 small handful of clover sprouts (optional)
1 lime, peeled if not organic

Cut the cucumber to fit your juicer's feed tube. Juice half the cucumber first. Bunch up the sprouts and wrap in one kale leaf and the spinach in the other kale leaf. Turn off the machine and add them. Turn the machine back on and push through slowly with the rest of the cucumber, then juice the remaining cucumber and lime. Stir ingredients, pour into a glass, and drink as soon as possible. Serves 1–2.

Super Green

1 green apple
4 kale leaves
2 ribs of celery with leaves
1 cucumber, peeled if not organic
1 lemon, peeled if not organic
1-inch-chunk of ginger

Cut produce to fit your juicer's feed tube. Start with apple, juice all ingredients, and stir. Pour into a glass and drink as soon as possible. Serves 2.

Super Sprout Drink

1 organic cucumber, scrubbed well
1 small handful of clover or radish sprouts
1 large handful of sunflower sprouts
1 small handful of buckwheat sprouts
2 kale leaves

Do not peel the organic cucumber. Cut produce to fit your juicer's feed tube. Wrap sprouts in kale leaves and push through juicer slowly. Juice ingredients and stir. Pour into a glass and drink as soon as possible. Serves 1.

Sweet Serenity

1 handful of spinach
1 romaine leaf
1 green apple
2 ribs of celery with leaves
1 cucumber, peeled if not organic
1 lime, peeled if not organic

Cut produce to fit your juicer's feed tube. Wrap spinach in the romaine leaf. Start with apple, then push the lettuce wrap through slowly, and follow with remaining ingredients and stir. Pour into a glass and drink as soon as possible. Serves 1.

Tomato and Spice

2 medium tomatoes
2 dark green leaves
1 small handful of parsley
1 lime or lemon, peeled if not organic
Dash of hot sauce

Cut produce to fit your juicer's feed tube. Juice all ingredients and stir. Pour into a glass and drink as soon as possible. Serves 1.

Tomato Florentine

2 tomatoes
4–5 sprigs of basil
1 large handful of spinach
1 lemon, peeled if not organic

Juice one tomato. Wrap the basil in several spinach leaves. Turn off the machine and add the spinach and basil. Turn the machine back on and gently tap to juice them. Juice the remaining tomato and lemon. Stir juice, pour into a glass and drink as soon as possible. Serves 1.

Totally Green

5 green leaf lettuce leaves
1 handful of parsley
1 handful of spinach
2 ribs of celery with leaves
1 green apple (for a little sweet taste)

Cut produce to fit your juicer's feed tube. Wrap the parsley and spinach in the lettuce leaves and push through the juicer slowly with the celery and apple. Stir the juice and drink as soon as possible. Serves 1.

Veggie Tonic

1 handful of spinach
1 dark green lettuce leaf
3 ribs of celery with leaves
2 ends of asparagus
1 large tomato
1 lemon, peeled

Cut produce to fit your juicer's feed tube. Wrap spinach in lettuce leaf and push through juicer slowly. Juice remaining ingredients and stir. Pour into a glass and drink as soon as possible. Serves 1.

Very Veggie Rejuvenator

½ tomato
1 cucumber, peeled if not organic
2 carrots, scrubbed well, tops removed, ends trimmed
2 ribs of celery with leaves
1 kale leaf
½ cup green cabbage
1 green onion

Cut produce to fit your juicer's feed tube. Juice all ingredients and stir. Pour into a glass and drink as soon as possible. Serves 2.

Wild Green Energy

1 cucumber, peeled if not organic
1 rib of celery with leaves
1 handful of wild greens such as dandelion, nettles, plantain, lamb's
    quarters, or sorrel
1 apple (green is lower in sugar)
1 lemon, peeled if not organic

Cut all ingredients to fit your juicer's feed tube and juice. Stir the
juice and drink as soon as possible. Serves 1.

Smoothies

Smoothies can be made in minutes, and you can quickly add a
variety of supplements such as vitamin C, barley greens, or bee
pollen. Many recipes incorporate greens and taste yummy (picky
eaters will never even know the greens are there). As you sip your
somewhat decadent shake, you'll know you're doing something
really good for your body, not just your taste buds.

Almond Swirl

1 cup almond milk
2 ripe peaches, pits removed, cut in chunks
½ cup kale, chopped
1–2 drops of stevia
1 tsp. pure vanilla extract
½ tsp. pure almond extract
6 ice cubes

Combine all ingredients in a blender and process well until
smooth and creamy. Serve chilled. Serves 2.

Avocado Cream

½ cup almond milk
1 avocado, peeled and pitted
1 handful of spinach
2 Tbsp. fresh lemon juice
2–3 drops of stevia
1 tsp. pure vanilla extract
1 tsp. freshly grated organic lemon peel
6 ice cubes

Combine all ingredients in a blender and process well until smooth and creamy. Serve chilled. Serves 1.

Berry Mania

½ cup almond milk
½ cup plain low-fat yogurt
½ cup chopped kale
½ cup loosely packed baby spinach
½ cup fresh or frozen blueberries
½ cup fresh or frozen raspberries
½ cup fresh or frozen blackberries
1 frozen banana, cut in chunks

Combine all ingredients in a blender and process well until smooth and creamy. Serve immediately. Serves 2.

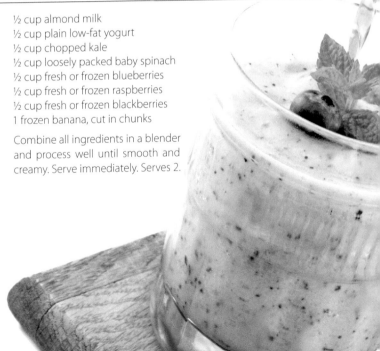

Berry Smooth

1 cup coconut milk
1 handful of spinach
2 cups fresh or frozen berries (blueberries, blackberries, or
    raspberries)
6 ice cubes (optional, may not be needed if using frozen fruit)

Pour the milk in a blender and add the spinach, berries, and ice; process until smooth and creamy. Serve as soon as possible. Serves 1.

Brain Power

½ cup plain yogurt
1 cup fresh or frozen strawberries, with caps
1 cup kale, chopped
½ cup orange juice
1 Tbsp. lecithin granules
1 Tbsp. protein powder of choice
1 tsp. pure vanilla extract
2–3 drops of stevia
6–8 ice cubes

Put all ingredients in a blender and process until smooth and creamy. Serve as soon as possible. Serves 1–2.

Cherie's Green Morning Blend

½ English cucumber, peeled and cut in chunks
1 avocado, peeled, pitted and cut in quarters
1 cup loosely packed baby spinach
Juice of 1 lime
1 Tbsp. green powder of choice (optional)
2–3 Tbsp. ground almonds (optional)

Combine ingredients in a blender and blend well. Sprinkle ground almonds on top, as desired. Serves 1.

Coconut Creamsicle

1 cup coconut milk
½ cup grated coconut, lightly packed
½ cup loosely packed baby spinach
2 tsp. pure vanilla extract
4–5 drops of stevia
6 ice cubes

Place all ingredients in a blender and process until smooth and creamy. Pour into glasses and serve chilled. Serves 2.

Coconut Green Delight

1 cucumber, cut in chunks
1 cup raw spinach, kale, or chard, chopped
1 avocado, peeled, seeded,
    and cut in quarters
½ cup coconut milk
1 Tbsp. organic virgin coconut oil
Juice of 1 lime or lemon

Combine all ingredients in a blender and
process until smooth. Serves 2.

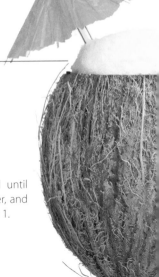

Cranberry-Pear Fat Buster

2 pears, Bartlett or Asian
1 cucumber, peeled if not organic
½ cup loosely packed baby spinach
¼ lemon, peeled if not organic
2 Tbsp. cranberries, fresh or frozen
½- to 1-inch-chunk of ginger
6 ice cubes (optional)

Chop up pears and cucumber and blend until smooth. Add lemon juice, cranberries, ginger, and ice as desired, and blend until creamy. Serves 1.

Dandelion Morning

½ bunch dandelion greens
2 ribs of celery with leaves
1-inch-chunk of fresh ginger
1 green apple
1 cup berries, fresh or frozen

Combine all ingredients in a blender and process until smooth and creamy. Serves 2.

Green Berry Blast

1 cucumber, peeled if not organic
½ green apple
1 cup berries (blueberries, raspberries, or blackberries) fresh, or frozen thawed
3–4 dark green leaves (collard, Swiss chard, or kale)
1-inch-chunk of ginger
Juice of ½ lemon
1 avocado, peeled, pitted, and cut in chunks

Cut the cucumber and apple in chunks. Place the cucumber, apple and berries in a blender and process until smooth. Chop the greens and ginger and add to the blender along with the juice of half a lemon and avocado and process until well blended. Serves 2.

Green Lemonade Slush

2 green apples
Juice of ½ lemon
1 handful of spinach
6–8 ice cubes

Place all ingredients in a blender and process until smooth. Pour into glasses and serve chilled. Serves 2.

Green Smoothie Supreme

    1 broccoli stem (save the florets for steaming, if you like)
    1 green apple
    1 lemon
    ½ cucumber, peeled if not organic, cut in chunks
    1 handful of spinach
    1 small handful of parsley
    1 cup blueberries (fresh or frozen)
    1 kiwi
    1 avocado, peeled, pitted, and cut in chunks
    2–3 drops of stevia
    4–6 ice cubes, as desired

Juice the broccoli stem, apple, and lemon. Pour the juice in the blender, and add the cucumber, spinach, parsley, blueberries, kiwi, and avocado. Add stevia if you like it sweeter and ice cubes if you like it cold. Blend until the mixture is smooth and creamy. Serves 2.

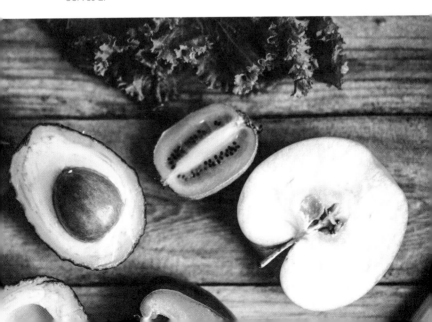

Healthy Green Smoothie

1 cucumber, peeled if not organic
2 ribs of celery
1 handful of kale, parsley, or spinach
1 green apple
½ lemon, peeled if not organic
6 ice cubes

Chop the cucumber, celery, greens, and apple. Place in blender with lemon and ice; process until creamy. Serves 2.

Muscle Power

Cashews and chard are rich in magnesium, which plays a critical role in converting carbohydrates to energy. This mineral also controls heartbeat and muscle contractions, and it is important for muscle relaxation and prevention of muscle spasms.

⅔ cup fresh apple juice (about 2 apples, juiced)
1 cup fresh or frozen strawberries (8–10 strawberries)
½ cup raw cashews
1 cup chopped chard
1 Tbsp. protein powder of choice
½ tsp. ascorbic acid (vitamin C powder)
6 ice cubes

Pour the apple juice into a blender and add the strawberries, cashews, protein powder, ascorbic acid, and ice. Blend on high speed until smooth and serve immediately. Serves 1.

Rockin' Berries

2 cups fresh or frozen berries (blueberries, blackberries, or
    raspberries)
1 cup almond or coconut milk
½ cup acai berry juice
1 tsp. pure vanilla extract
6 ice cubes (optional, may not be needed if using frozen fruit)

Combine the milk in a blender with the berries, juice, vanilla, and
ice. Blend until smooth and creamy. Serves 1.

Spicy Tomato

5 tomatoes, chopped
1 cucumber, peeled if not organic
3 ribs of celery, cut in chunks
1 kale leaf, chopped
1 garlic clove, peeled, chopped
Dash of kelp powder or dulse flakes
1 avocado, peeled, pitted, cut in chunks

Combine tomatoes in blender and process on low. Add
cucumber and continue to blend on low, then add celery and
blend on high quickly. Add a bit of water if mixture becomes
too thick. Next add kale leaf, garlic, and kelp or dulse, and blend
mixture on high. Add avocado and blend on high until well
mixed. Serves 2.

Sprouted Almond-Vanilla Smoothie

1 cup raw almonds
1 cup unsweetened almond milk
1 cup berries of choice
½ tsp. pure vanilla extract
6 ice cubes

Soak almonds in purified water overnight so that they will sprout. (Sprouting allows the almond to partially germinate, which removes the enzyme inhibitors and increases nutrient value.) Blend together almonds, almond milk, berries, vanilla, and ice. Pour in glasses and serve as soon as possible. Serves 2.

Sugar-Free Green Smoothie

1 cup plain yogurt
1 large handful of spinach
1 kale leaf, chopped
1 Tbsp. tahini (sesame butter)
1 tsp. pure raspberry extract
1 tsp. pure vanilla extract
½ tsp. freshly grated organic orange peel
1–2 drops of stevia (optional)
6 ice cubes

Place all ingredients in blender and process until creamy and smooth. Serve chilled. Serves 1.

Sunday Brunch

2 tomatoes, chopped
1 handful of cilantro, chopped
Juice of 1 lime
Pinch of Celtic sea salt
Dash of hot sauce

Combine all ingredients in blender and process until creamy and smooth. Serve chilled. Serves 2.

Super Green Smoothie

1¼ cups fresh cucumber juice (about 1 large or 2 medium
    cucumbers, peeled if not organic)
2 ribs of celery with leaves, juiced
1 kale leaf, chopped
1 avocado, peeled, seeded, and cut in chunks
1 garlic clove, peeled
4 ounces soft silken organic tofu
½ cup flat-leaf parsley, coarsely chopped
2 tsp. sweet onion, minced
1 tsp. dried dill weed

Pour the cucumber and celery juices into a blender and add the
kale, avocado, garlic, tofu, parsley, onion, and dill. Blend on high
speed until smooth and creamy; serve immediately as it does
not taste good if it sits. Serves 2.

Sweet Dandelion Smoothie

1 pear, Bartlett or Asian
1 apple (green has less sugar)
1 large handful of dandelion greens
1-inch-chunk gingerroot
1 cup coconut milk
Juice of ½ lemon
¼ cup flaxseeds
6 ice cubes (optional)

Place all ingredients in a blender and process until it becomes a
creamy shake. Serves 2.

Tomato-Lemon-Cucumber-Avocado

2 tomatoes, cut in chunks
1 cucumber, peeled if not organic, cut in chunks
Juice of 1 lemon
1 handful of cilantro
1 avocado, peeled and pitted, cut in chunks

Place all ingredients in a blender and blend until smooth. Pour in glasses and serve chilled. Serves 2.

Tomato-Lemon Twister

2 tomatoes, cut in chunks, frozen
1 cup tomato juice (2–3 medium tomatoes, juiced)
½ cup packed baby spinach
Juice of 1 lemon
1 tsp. freshly grated lemon rind, organic
6 fresh basil leaves, rinsed

Place the tomato chunks in a freezer bag and freeze them until solid. Pour the tomato juice into a blender and add the frozen tomato chunks, spinach, lemon juice, lemon peel, and basil. Blend on high speed until smooth and serve immediately. Serves 2.

Top of the Mornin'

½ cup almond milk
1 cup plain low-fat yogurt
1 cup frozen peaches, cut in chunks
1 cup frozen blueberries
½ cup packed baby spinach
4–5 drops of stevia
1 tsp. pure vanilla extract

Place all ingredients in a blender and process until smooth and creamy. Pour in glasses, sprinkle ground almonds or chia seeds on top, and serve chilled. Serves 2.

Weight-Loss Partner

1 cup coconut milk
1 cup berries of choice
½ cup packed baby spinach
1–2 Tbsp. protein powder of choice
1 Tbsp. virgin organic coconut oil
1 Tbsp. ground flax seeds
1 tsp. pure vanilla extract
¼ tsp. almond extract
2–3 drops of stevia
6–8 ice cubes

Combine all ingredients but ice in a blender and process until creamy and smooth. Add ice after the coconut oil is blended so that it won't clump. You may use more or less ice, depending on how cold you like your smoothie. Serves 1–2.

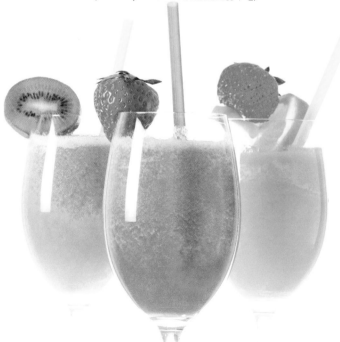

Appendix A

HELPFUL FOODS FOR
DIABETIC MENU-PLANNING

S EE THE RECIPES throughout this book for novel and delicious ways to combine these foods. You will be surprised how many of these foods can be juiced.[1]

Vegetables

Low in carbohydrates (includes only the vegetables mentioned in this book; there are many others that are good for you):

- Artichoke, Jerusalem

- Asparagus

- Beans (green, wax, Italian)

- Brussels sprouts

- Broccoli

- Cabbage (all types)

- Celery

- Cucumber

- Fennel

- Greens (beet, collard, kale, mustard, turnip)

- Jicama

- Kohlrabi, kohlrabi greens

- Onions

- Peppers (all types)

- Radishes
- Salad greens (arugula, chicory, dandelion, endive, escarole, lettuce, parsley, radicchio, romaine, spinach, watercress, wild greens)
- Sprouts (all types)
- Summer squash (all types)
- Spinach
- Swiss chard
- Tomatoes

Higher in carbohydrates:

- Beets
- Corn
- Peas
- Potato (sweet or white, baked)
- Yams
- Winter squash

Fruits

- Apples (green are lower in sugar)
- Applesauce (no sugar added)
- Avocados
- Blackberries, blueberries
- Cantaloupe
- Currants, black
- Cherries
- Elderberries

- Grapefruit
- Kiwi
- Lemon
- Lime
- Mangoes
- Peaches
- Pears
- Plums
- Quinces
- Raspberries
- Strawberries

Higher glycemic load, most other fruits, including:

- Bananas
- Melons
- Oranges
- Tangerines
- Watermelon
- Dates, raisins, figs, prunes, other dried fruits

Other foods

- Whole grains, whole-grain cereals
- Baked goods made with whole-grain flours, whole rye flour, buckwheat flour
- Basil, cilantro, spearmint
- Corn, popcorn, corn tortillas, and other products made from organic corn

- Whole oats/oatmeal
- Quinoa, millet, grain sorghum (milo), triticale
- Barley
- Bulgur (cracked wheat)
- Brown, black, red rice, wild rice
- Lower-fat cuts of meat or fish (not fried)
- Tofu (not fried)
- Dried beans and peas (e.g., pinto, lima, black beans; black-eyed and split green peas)
- Sugar-free baked beans
- Fat-free refried beans
- Lentils
- Pastured or free-range eggs
- Nuts and seeds (e.g., almonds, cashews, walnuts, chia seeds, flax seeds)
- Animal protein: wild-caught fish, free-range or pastured chicken, grass-fed beef

Appendix B

GLYCEMIC INDEX, GLYCEMIC LOAD

WHICH IS MORE useful to your diabetic meal-planning? Glycemic index (GI) or glycemic load (GL)?[1]

GI numbers can be deceiving, because they do not take into account portion size. The GI has been developed by researchers, and they calculate it from servings that contained 50 grams of carbohydrate. This is not a realistic serving size for many vegetables and fruits. (For example, you would have to eat 1½ pounds of carrots to get 50 grams of carbohydrate, so although carrots have a GI that is relatively high for a vegetable (71), a half-cup serving has a GL of less than 6!)

The GL is determined by multiplying the number of grams of carbohydrate in a serving (8 grams per ½ cup of carrots) by the GI of the food, as a percentage:

- 8 grams of carbohydrates per half cup x .71 (71 being the GI of carrots) = 5.68

- Low-GL foods are those that rank less than 10 or 11.

- Moderate-GL foods are those that rank between 11 and 19.

- High-GL foods are those that rank higher than 20.

Sample glycemic load charts can be found online by searching for "glycemic load."[2]

NOTES

Introduction

1. Centers for Disease Control and Prevention, *National Diabetes Statistics Report: Estimates of Diabetes and Its Burden in the United States, 2014* (Atlanta, GA: US Department of Health and Human Services, 2014), accessed February 11, 2016, http://www.cdc.gov/diabetes/pubs/statsreport14/national-diabetes-report-web.pdf.

2. Ibid.

Chapter 2—Diabetes and You

1. These symptoms (and more) are detailed in many places. One online source of information is Harvard's Joslin Diabetes Center http://www.joslin.org/info/general_diabetes_facts_and_information.html.

2. The information about diabetes within quotation marks comes from the *National Diabetes Statistics Report: Estimates of Diabetes and Its Burden in the United States, 2014*, Centers for Disease Control and Prevention.

3. Ibid.

4. Veronika Charvatova, "Diabetes Fact Sheet," Viva!, accessed February 12, 2016, http://www.viva.org.uk/diabetes-fact-sheet.

5. "Eat Right!", Centers for Disease Control and Prevention, accessed February 12, 2016, http://www.cdc.gov/diabetes/managing/eatright.html.

6. F. Andreelii et al., "What Can Bariatric Surgery Teach Us About the Pathophysiology of Type 2 Diabetes?", Diabetes & Metabolism. 35, no. 6 (2009): 499–507.

7. "Eat Right!", Centers for Disease Control and Prevention.

8. "Counting Carbs? Understanding Glycemic Index and Glycemic Load," NIH News in Health, December 2012, accessed February 15, 2016, http://newsinhealth.nih.gov/issue/Dec2012/Feature2.

9. "Glycemic Index and Diabetes," American Diabetes Association, accessed November 4, 2015, http://www.diabetes.org/food-and-fitness/food/what-can-i-eat/understanding-carbohydrates/glycemic-index-and-diabetes.html.

10. Ibid.

11. Nina K., "Are Green Apples Better Than Red on Low-Carb Diets?" December 18, 2013, Healthy Eating, Livestrong.com, accessed November 4, 2015, http://www.livestrong.com/article/357142-are-green-apples-better-on-low-carb-diets-than-red/.

12. Survey adapted from Health24; see more at http://www.feelgoodhealth.co.za/health-hub/

lose-weight-insulin-resistance-diabetes-fatigue-mood-swings#sthash
.ycAWHriD.dpuf), as posted on my website, Cherie Calbom: The Juice
Lady, http://www.juiceladycherie.com/Juice/take-the-insulin-resistance
-quiz/.

Chapter 3—The Importance of Losing Weight

1. J. Tuomilehto et al., "Prevention of Type 2 Diabetes Mellitus by Changes
   in Lifestyle Among Subjects With Impaired Glucose Tolerance," *New
   England Journal of Medicine* 344 (2001): 1343–1350; "Reduction
   in the Incidence of Type 2 Diabetes With Lifestyle Intervention or Met-
   formin," *New England Journal of Medicine* 346 (2003): 393–403;
   Marion J. Franz, "The Dilemma of Weight Loss in Diabetes," *Diabetes
   Spectrum* 20, no. 3 (2007): 133–136, accessed July 2, 2015, http://
   spectrum.diabetesjournals.org/content/20/3/133.full.

2. Franz, "The Dilemma of Weight Loss in Diabetes."

3. "Will Weight Loss Help Your Diabetes?", WebMD, accessed February 16,
   2016, http://www.webmd.com/diabetes/safe-diet-tips-for-diabetes.

4. Ibid.

5. "Insulin and Weight Gain: Keep the Pounds Off," Mayo Clinic, August 19,
   2014, accessed Nov. 4, 2015, www.mayoclinic.org/diseases-conditions
   /diabetes/in-depth/insulin-and-weight-gain/art-20047836.

6. Ibid.

7. "NWCR Facts" National Weight Control Registry, accessed February 16,
   2016, www.nwcr.ws/Research/default.htm.

8. "Dr. Oz's Top 5 Mistakes Dieters Make," posted by Donny Osmond Radio,
   donny.com, accessed February 16, 2016, http://donny.com/radio-posts
   /dr-ozs-top-5-mistakes-dieters-make/.

9. Judy Siegel, "Garlic Prevents Obesity," *Jerusalem Post*, October 30,
   2001, 5.

10. Franz, "The Dilemma of Weight Loss in Diabetes."

11. "Vegetable Juice May Help With Weight Loss," Reuters.com, April 22,
    2009, accessed February 5, 2010, www.reuters.com/article
    /idUSTRE53L60S20090422.

12. Ibid.

13. "Vegetable Use Aided in Dietary Support for Weight Loss and Lower
    Blood Pressure," MedicalNewsToday.com, October 21, 2009, accessed
    February 5, 2010, www.medicalnewstoday.com/articles/168174.php.

14. Ibid.

15. Ibid.; "What Is Metabolic Syndrome?" WebMD.com, accessed February
    16, 2016, www.webmd.com/heart/metabolic-syndrome/metabolic
    -syndrome-what-is-it.

16. "What Is Metabolic Syndrome?" WebMD.com

17. R. Akilen et al., "Glycated Haemoglobin and Blood Pressure-Lowering Effect of Cinnamon in Multi-EthnicType 2 Diabetic Patients in the UL: A Randomized, Placebo-Controlled, Double-Blind Clinical Trial," *Diabetic Medicine* 27, no. 10 (October 2010): 1159–1167.

18. Nanci Hellmich, "Sleep Loss (May) = Weight Gain: Healthy Weight Might Rest With Diet, Exercise and Sleep-Linked Hormones," *USA Today*, December 7, 2004, accessed February 16, 2016, www.usatoday.com/educate/college/healthscience/articles/20041212.htm.

19. James E. Gangwisch et al., "Inadequate Sleep as a Risk Factor for Obesity: Analyses of the NHANES I," *Sleep* 28, no. 10 (2005): 1289–1296.

20. Colette Bouchez, "The Dream Diet: Losing Weight While You Sleep," Healthy Sleep Texas, accessed February 16, 2016, http://www.healthysleeptexas.com/2012/02/the-dream-diet-losing-weight-while-you-sleep/.

21. John Easton, "Lack of Sleep Alters Hormones, Metabolism," *University of Chicago Chronicle*, December 2, 1999, accessed February 16, 2016, http://chronicle.uchicago.edu/991202/sleep.shtml.

22. Bouchez, "The Dream Diet: Losing Weight While You Sleep."

23. Ibid.

24. Easton, "Lack of Sleep Alters Hormones, Metabolism."

25. Cherie Calbom and John Calbom, *Sleep Away the Pounds* (New York: Warner Wellness, 2007).

Chapter 4—Ditch the Sugar

1. The first part of this chapter has been modified from several of my blog posts, notably "Sugar and Inflammation," www.juiceladycherie.com/Juice/sugar-and-inflammation, and "8 Reasons to Ditch Sugar," www.juiceladycherie.com/Juice/8-reasons-to-ditch-sugar, accessed February 16, 2016.

2. Byron Richards, "High Fructose Corn Syrup Makes Your Brain Crave Food," Wellness Resoures, April 2, 2009, accessed February 16, 2016, http://www.wellnessresources.com/weight/articles/high_fructose_corn_syrup_makes_your_brain_crave_food/.

3. Yoshio Nagai et al., "The Role of Peroxisome Proliferator-Activated Receptor Coactivator-1 in the Pathogenesis of Fructose-Induced Insulin Resistance," *Cell Metabolism* 9, no. 3 (March 4, 2009): 252–264.

4. Alice Park, "Can Sugar Substitutes Make You Fat?" *Time*, February 10, 2008, accessed February 16, 2016, http://content.time.com/time/health/article/0,8599,1711763,00.html.

5. Cherie Calbom, "The Dangers of Aspartame—Part II," March 29, 2013, accessed February 16, 2016, http://www.juiceladycherie.com/Juice/the -dangers-of-aspartame-part-ii/, information provided by H. J. Roberts, Palm Beach Institute for Medical Research, Inc.

6. "Blueberries May Help Reduce Belly Fat, Diabetes Risk," ScienceDaily .com, April 20, 2009, accessed February 16, 2016, http:// www.sciencedaily.com/releases/2009/04/090419170112.htm.

7. Richard Fogoros, "Low Glycemic Weight Loss Is Longer Lasting," About .com, January 3, 2005, accessed February 16, 2016, http://heartdisease .about.com/od/dietandobesity/a/logly.htm.

8. Jennie Brand-Miller, "A Glycemic Index Expert Responds to the Tufts Research," DiabetesHealth.com, accessed February 16, 2016, www .diabeteshealth.com/a-glycemic-index-expert-responds-to-the-tufts -research/.

9. Mark Hyman, "How Toxins Make You Fat: 4 Steps to Get Rid of Toxic Weight," October 18, 2014, accessed February 16, 2016, http://drhyman .com/blog/2012/02/20/how-toxins-make-you-fat-4-steps-to-get-rid-of -toxic-weight/#close.

10. Ibid.; O. A. Jones, M. L. Maguire, J. L. Griffin, "Environmental Pollu- tion and Diabetes: A Neglected Association," *Lancet* 371, no. 9609 (Jan- uary 26, 2008): 287–288.

11. Hyman, "How Toxins Make You Fat: 4 Steps to Get Rid of Toxic Weight,"

12. "Industrial Pollution Doesn't Have to Begin in The Womb," Environ- mental Working Group, accessed February 16, 2016, http://www.ewg .org/enviroblog/2009/02/industrial-pollution-doesnt-have-begin-womb; Hyman, "How Toxins Make You Fat: 4 Steps to Get Rid of Toxic Weight."

13. Get an overview of detoxing on my website at www.juiceladycherie.com /Juice/cleansing-detoxification/.

Chapter 5—Why Juice?

1. Wang, Hong, et al. "Total Antioxidant Capacity of Fruits" *Journal of Agricultural and Food Chemistry* 44 (1996): 701–705.

2. First for Women, "Dr. Oz's #1 Fat Cure," January 10, 2011, 32–35.

3. Adein Cassidy et al., "Plasma Adiponectin Concentrations Are Associ- ated With Body Composition and Plant-Based Dietary Factors in Female Twins," *Journal of Nutrition* 139, no. 2 (February 2009): 353–358.

4. Diane Feskanich et al., "Vitamin K Intake and Hip Fractures in Women: A Prospective Study," American Journal of Clinical Nutrition 69, no. 1 (January 1999): 74–79, accessed February 16, 2016, http://www.ajcn .org/content/69/1/74.full.

5. Patrice Carter et al., "Fruit and Vegetable Intake and Incidence of Type 2 Diabetes Millitus: Systematic Review and Meta-Analysis," *British Medical Journal* 341 (August 2010), accessed February http://www.bmj .com/content/341/bmj.c4229.full.

6. T. Kondo et al., Vinegar Intake Reduces Body Weight, Body Fat Mass, and Serum Triglyceride Levels in Obese Japanese Subjects," *Bioscience, Biotechnology, and Biochemistry* 73, no. 8 (August 2009), accessed February 16, 2016, http://www.ncbi.nlm.nih.gov/pubmed/19661687.

7. Michelle Pellizzon, "3 Metabolism-Boosting Tonics to Help You Burn Calories All Day Long," Thrive Market, December 8, 2015, accessed February 16, 2016, http://tinyurl.com/zmdlbfh.

8. Brindusa Vanta, "The Benefits of Wheatgrass for Diabetes," February 2, 2014, Livestrong, accessed February 16, 2016, http://www.livestrong .com/article/367210-the-benefits-of-wheatgrass-for-diabetes.

9. Ibid.

10. Ibid.

Chapter 6—Living Foods Make All the Difference in Diabetes

1. See, for example, the article and video documentary "Type 2 Diabetes Cure," Raw Foods, Living Foods, accessed February 16, 2016, http:// www.rawfoods-livingfoods.com/type-2-diabetes-cure.html.

2. "New Analysis Suggests 'Diet Soda Paradox'—Less Sugar, More Weight," UT Health Science Center San Antonio news release, June 14, 2005, accessed February 16, 2016, http://www.uthscsa.edu/hscnews /singleformat2.asp?newID=1539.

3. Joseph Mercola, "McDonald's and Biophoton Deficiency," Mercola.com, August 21, 2002 accessed February 16, 2016, http://articles.mercola .com/sites/articles/archive/2002/08/21/biophoton.aspx.

4. John Switzer, "Bio-Photon Nutrition and Wild Green Energy Cocktails for Optimal Health (English)," May 21, 2009, accessed February 16, 2016, http://ein-langes-leben.de/raw-food-english/bio-photon-nutrition -and-wild-energy-cocktails-for-optimal-health-english.

5. "Light Affects Nutrients," PCC Sound Consumer, March 2012, accessed February 16, 2016, http://www.pccnaturalmarkets.com/sc/1203/light _nutrients.html.

6. Virginia Worthington, "Nutritional Quality of Organic Versus Conventional Fruits, Vegetables, and Grains," *Journal of Alternative and Complementary Medicine* 7, no. 2 (2001): 161–173.

7. "Official: Organic Really Is Better," TimesOnline.co.uk, October 28, 2007.

8. Tara Parker-Pope, "Five Easy Ways to Go Organic," *New York Times*, October 22, 2007, accessed February 16, 2016, http://well.blogs.nytimes .com/2007/10/22/five-easy-ways-to-go-organic/.

9. Ibid.

Chapter 7—Helpful Recipes for Diabetes— Juices and Smoothies

1. Dae Jung Kim, et al., "Magnesium Intake in Relation to Systemic Inflammation, Insulin Resistance, and the Incidence of Diabetes," *Diabetes Care* 33, no. 12 (December 2010): 2604–2610.

Appendix A—Beneficial Foods for Diabetic Menu-Planning

1. This list was compiled from several sources, including "Grains and Starchy Vegetables," American Diabetes Association, http://www .diabetes.org/food-and-fitness/food/what-can-i-eat/making-healthy-food -choices/grains-and-starchy-vegetables.html; "Non-Starchy Vegetables," American Diabetes Association, accessed February 16, 2016, http://www .diabetes.org/food-and-fitness/food/what-can-i-eat/making-healthy-food -choices/non-starchy-vegetables.html; "Best and Worst Foods for Diabetes" WebMD, accessed February 16, 2016, www.webmd.com/diabetes /diabetic-food-list-best-worst-foods; and online glycemic load charts.

Appendix B: Glycemic Index, Glycemic Load

1. From Amy Campbell, "Glycemic Index and Glycemic Load," Diabetes Self-Management, August 28, 2006, accessed February 16, 2016, www .diabetesselfmanagement.com/blog/glycemic-index-and-glycemic-load, and "Estimated Glycemic Load," SELFNutritionData, accessed February 16, 2016, http://nutritiondata.self.com/help/estimated-glycemic-load. See also "Glycemic Index Defined" and "Glycemic Load Defined," Glycemic Research Institute, accessed February 16, 2016, http://www.glycemic .com/GlycemicIndex-LoadDefined.htm.

2. For example, "Glycemic Index and Glycemic Load for 100+ Foods," Harvard Medical School Health Publications, http://www.health.harvard .edu/healthy-eating/glycemic_index_and_glycemic_load_for_100_foods.

FOR MORE INFORMATION

The Juice Lady's Juicy Tips Newsletter

Sign up for free at www.juiceladyinfo.com.

Cherie's Websites

www.juiceladyinfo.com, www.juiceladycherie.com, or www
.cheriecalbom.com—information on juicing and weight loss

The Juice Lady's Health and Wellness Juice Cleanse Retreats

I invite you to join us for a week that can change your life!
Our retreats offer gourmet organic raw foods with a three-day
juice fast midweek. We present interesting, informative classes
in a beautiful, peaceful setting where you can experience healing
and restoration of body and soul. For more information and dates
for the retreats, visit www.juiceladycherie.com/Juice/juice-raw
-food-retreat/ or call 866-8GETWEL (866-843-8935).

The Juice Lady's Jumpstart Health and Fitness 8-Week E-Course

This 8-week e-course helps you achieve your health and fitness goals. I lead you step by step to better health and fitness.
I want you to embrace your own healthy lifestyle that you can
stick with for life. For more information, go to www.juicelady
cherie.com/Juice/healthy-and-fit-for-life/ or call 866-8GETWEL
(866-843-8935).

The Juice Lady's 30-Day Detox Challenge

This is a 4-week e-course designed to help your body get
rid of toxins, contaminants, waste, and heavy metals that can
accumulate in joints, organs, tissues, cells, the lymphatic system,
and the bloodstream. It can energize your entire body. For more

information, go to www.juiceladycherie.com/Juice/30-day-detox/ or call 866-8GETWEL (866-843-8935).

Healthy Holiday Cooking, Juicing, and Entertaining in Style 4-Week E-Course

This class is designed to help you navigate through the holiday season with healthy choices and keep your waistline. Weekly you'll get recipes and health tips plus ideas to overcome emotional eating. Enjoy "Yummy Juices, Treats, Appetizers, and Main Dishes."

Nutrition Consultation

To schedule a nutrition consultation with the Juice Lady's team, visit www.juiceladycherie.com/Juice/nutritional-counseling/ or call 866-8GETWEL (866-843-8935).

Scheduling Cherie Calbom to Speak

To schedule Cherie Calbom to speak for your organization, call 866-8GETWEL (866-843-8935).

Books by Cherie and John Calbom

These books can be ordered at any of the websites above or by calling 866-8GETWEL (866-843-8935).

- Cherie Calbom with Abby Fammartino, *The Juice Lady's Anti-Inflammation Diet* (Siloam)
- Cherie Calbom, *The Juice Lady's Big Book of Juices and Green Smoothies* (Siloam)
- Cherie Calbom, *The Juice Lady's Remedies for Asthma and Allergies* (Siloam)
- Cherie Calbom, *The Juice Lady's Remedies for Stress and Adrenal Fatigue* (Siloam)

- Cherie Calbom, *The Juice Lady's Remedies for Thyroid Disorders* (Siloam)

- Cherie Calbom, *The Juice Lady's Weekend Weight-Loss Diet* (Siloam)

- Cherie Calbom, *The Juice Lady's Living Foods Revolution* (Siloam)

- Cherie Calbom, *The Juice Lady's Turbo Diet* (Siloam)

- Cherie Calbom, *The Juice Lady's Guide to Juicing for Health* (Avery)

- Cherie Calbom and John Calbom, *Juicing, Fasting, and Detoxing for Life* (Wellness Central)

- Cherie Calbom, *The Wrinkle Cleanse* (Avery)

- Cherie Calbom and John Calbom, *The Coconut Diet* (Wellness Central)

- Cherie Calbom, John Calbom, and Michael Mahaffey, *The Complete Cancer Cleanse* (Thomas Nelson)

- Cherie Calbom, *The Ultimate Smoothie Book* (Wellness Central)

- Cherie Calbom, *The Juice Lady's Sugar Knockout* (Siloam)

Juicers

To find out about the best juicers recommended by Cherie, call 866-8GETWEL (866-843-8935) or visit www.juiceladyinfo.com.

Dehydrators

To find out the best dehydrators recommended by Cherie, call 866-8GETWEL (866-843-8935) or visit www.juiceladyinfo.com.

Lymphasizer

To view the Swing Machine (lymphasizer), visit www.juicelady-info.com or call 866-8GETWEL (866-843-8935).

Veggie Powders and Supplements

To purchase or get information on Wheatgrass Juice Powder, Barley Max, Carrot Juice Max, and Beet Max powders, go to www.juiceladyinfo.com or call 866-8GETWEL (866-843-8935). (These powders are ideal for when you travel or when you can't get juice.)

Internal Cleansing Kits

The complete and comprehensive internal cleansing kit contains eighteen items for a twenty-one-day cleanse program. You will receive a free colon cleanse kit, along with Liver-Gallbladder Rejuvenator, Friendly Bacteria Replenisher, Parasite Cleanser, Lung Rejuvenator, Kidney and Bladder Rejuvenator, Blood and Skin Rejuvenator, and Lymph Rejuvenator. See the website for more information.

You may order the cleansing products and get the 10 percent discount by calling 866-8GETWEL (866-843-8935).

BerryBreeze

Keep your produce fresher longer and your fridge smelling fresh too. It can save you up to $2,200 a year from lost produce. Go to www.juiceladycherie.com.

CONNECT WITH US!

CHARISMA HOUSE

(Spiritual Growth)

Facebook.com/CharismaHouse

@CharismaHouse

Instagram.com/CharismaHouseBooks

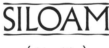

SILOAM

(Health)

Pinterest.com/CharismaHouse

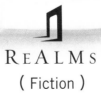

REALMS

(Fiction)

Facebook.com/RealmsFiction